The Ultimate Dandelion Medicine Book

40 Recipes for Using
Dandelion Leaves, Flowers, Stems, & Roots
as Medicine

CW01497747

Kristina Seleshanko

Table of Contents

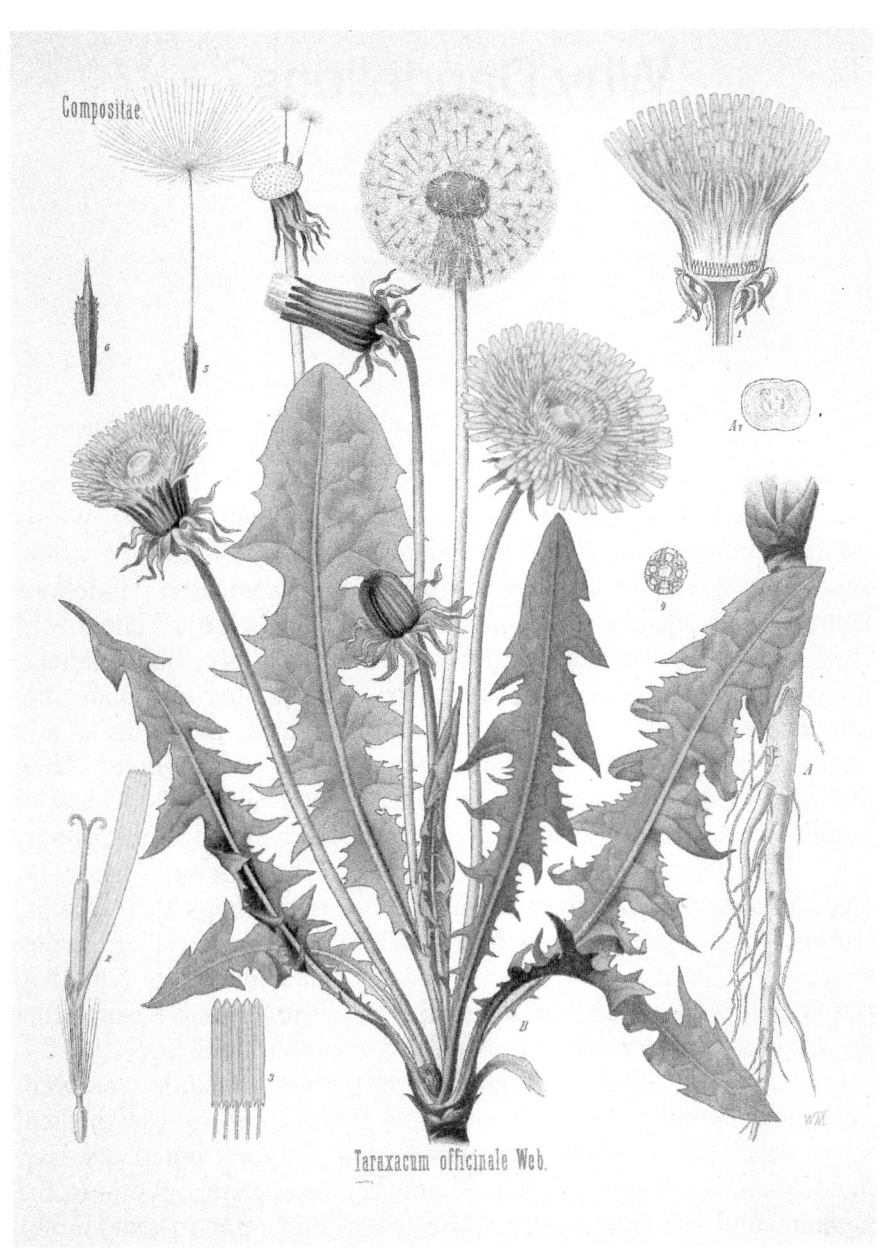

Compositae.

Taraxacum officinale Web.

Why Dandelions?

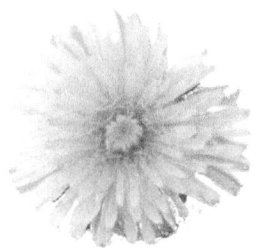

"Dandelion is, I'm convinced, one of the great tonic herbs of all times."
Herbalist Rosemary Gladstar

Americans mostly consider dandelions pesky weeds requiring eradication. They are a nuisance, at best, and at worst, something to use the strongest chemicals on. (Ironically, dandelions naturally help cleanse the body of exactly this type of chemical.) They invade our gardens and lawns in such a bright, bold manner, every neighbor notices them. They are, perhaps, the one plant that tells everyone who drives by our homes how much time and attention we put into our yards. (Dandelions everywhere? Then common wisdom says you must either be too lazy or too busy to garden.) They are the flower children love, but adults grumble about.

Yet it hasn't always been this way. The common dandelion isn't native to North America; our ancestors (perhaps the Vikings, perhaps later settlers) brought dandelion seeds with them when immigrating here - and they didn't do it accidentally. No, they secreted dandelion seeds among their few possessions because the plant is highly nutritious food that's also excellent medicine.

The first time the medicinal properties of dandelions were mentioned in written records was 659 B.C., in a Chinese medical book. Later, in the 10th century, Arab doctors noted its use. Dandelions were also used as medicine by the ancient Egyptians, the Romans, and the Greeks. Even the Bible may refer to dandelions, when, in the book of Exodus, it gives Passover instructions including the eating of "bitter herbs."

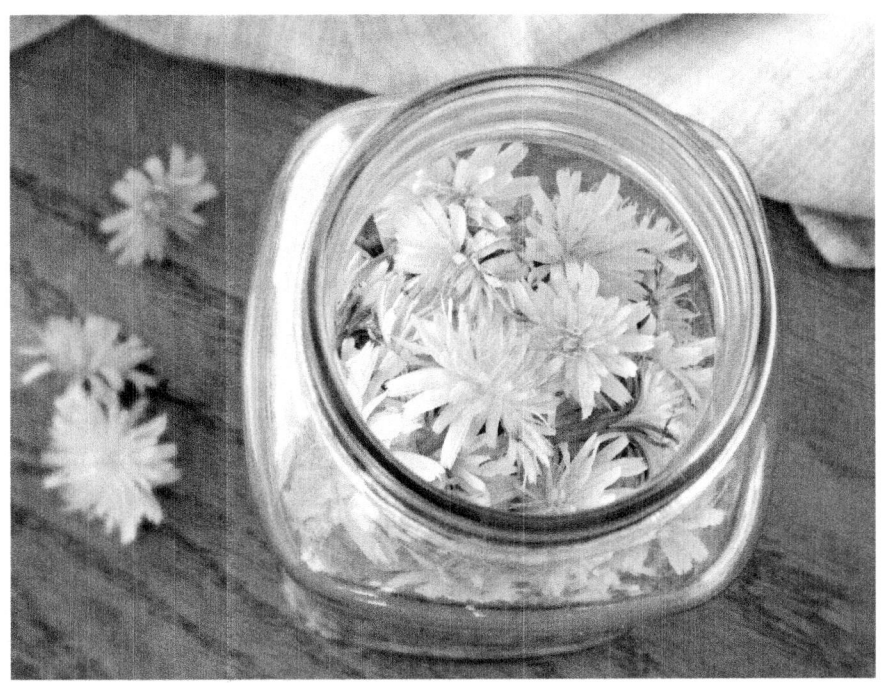

After that, nearly every culture where dandelions grew (the plant is currently on every continent but Antarctica) felt the weed important enough to include it in its medical literature.

In North America, native cultures readily embraced dandelions - not only as an abundant food source, but as a respected medicine. The Algonquians used them in poultices and ate the leaves for their medicinal properties. The Mohegans used dandelions for liver complaints (still considered the plant's most important medicinal use). The Cherokee used the root as a calming agent. The Aleut used dandelion leaves for sore throats. The Kiowa and Papago used dandelion flowers as a treatment for menstrual cramps. The Navajo used the root tea to help hasten the expulsion of the placenta after birth. The Iroquois used dandelions for jaundice and consumed a tea of the entire plant as a tonic. The Tewa made a poultice of the leaves for broken bones, swelling, and bruises. The Bella Coola used the roots to help cure gastrointestinal problems.

Even the dandelion's proper name tells us of its important medicinal history: *Taraxacum officinale*. *Taraxacum* means "bitter herb" (which references not just the plant's flavor, but its health qualities). This may be derived from the Greek *taraxos*, meaning "disorder remedy." *Officinale* is a term used to indicate plants with medicinal properties - specifically plants that were the official medicine of Roman apothecaries. (The plant's modern, common name - dandelion - is probably a mispronunciation of the French for "lion's teeth," or "dent de lion," which the dandelions leaves resemble.)

There are still other reasons not to destroy the dandelions growing in our yards: Not only are they good food and medicine for humans, but they do good things for nature. Their long roots, which can become as big as a large parsnip, do a fantastic job of aerating and draining the soil, as well as bringing nutrients that are deep in the earth nearer the surface (thereby increasing fertility for nearby plants with less aggressive root systems). This not only improves the soil, but it attracts earthworms, who also work hard to make the soil a better place for plants to grow.

Too, dandelions are a favorite among animals. Bees love to forage dandelion flowers. (In many cases, dandelions are their earliest and most prolific food.) And numerous wild animals - from elk and bear to porcupines and geese - use the plant for nourishing food.

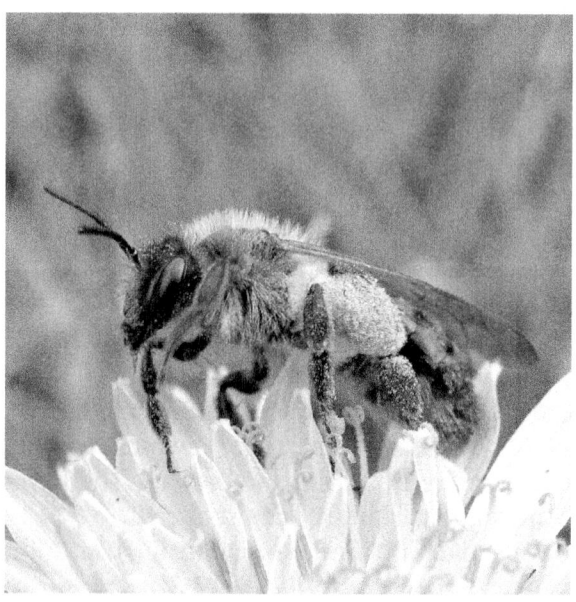

The response I've received from *The Ultimate Dandelion Cookbook* is remarkable. Some readers remember their grandparents using dandelions for food and medicine, and others, turned off by commercial foods low in nutrients and high in chemicals, are eager to learn the ways of their ancestors. Encouraged by the reaction to that cookbook, today I offer up more helpful tips for using dandelions - this time, as medicine.

The moment is ripe to learn about "the old ways." No, I don't believe modern medicine needs replacing with old. I, personally, am thankful for modern medical skill and knowledge. However, I believe our society is on the cusp of understanding that our ancestors were on to something when they pursued plants for healing. Though there's still much scientific research needed in the area of herbal medication (sadly, not a high priority because it's difficult to make billions of dollars selling an herb), some scientists and doctors have open minds about their use, encouraged by the scientific studies that bolster traditional claims (see the "Sampling of Scientific Studies Supporting Dandelion Medicine" section at the end of the book for a brief overview of them) and the improvement they see in their patients who do implement herbal medicine alongside conventional treatment.

I believe dandelions are the perfect introduction to herbal medicine. Nearly everyone has free and easy access to them, and most people can already identify them. So with a spirit of wonder at the resources God has supplied, I hope you'll do more than enjoy this book; I hope you will apply its information to your life and discover the joys of "dandy medicine."

Kristina

P.S. Do you love the idea of getting healthy, wild, free food and medicine? Check out the "Foraging" and "Herbs" sections on my blog: www.ProverbsThirtyOneWoman.blogspot.com.

Dandelions as Medicine

While there are some scientific studies about dandelions as medicine, most of them were conducted only on animals. Therefore, this book uses a mixture of tradition, animal studies, and personal experience when suggesting this plant for health. See the back of the book for references to scientific studies supporting the use of dandelions as medicine.

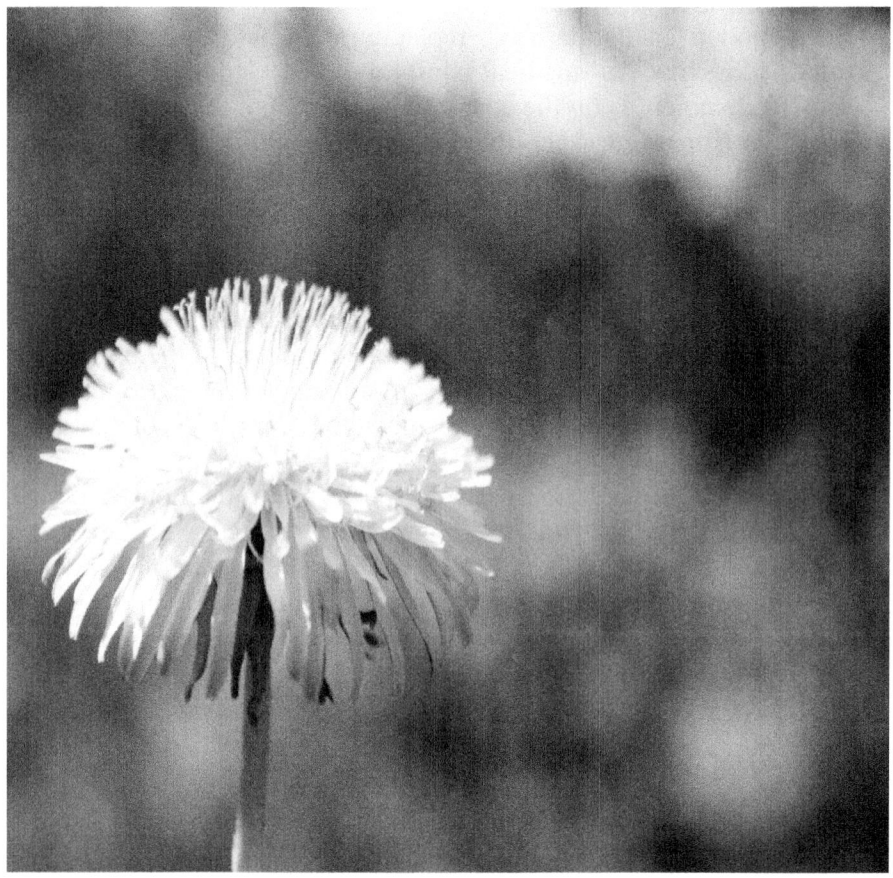

	Leaves	Flowers	Stems	Roots
Acne	x			x
Age spots		x		
Alzheimer's	x	x		x
Antifungal	x		x	x
Antimicrobial	x			x
Antioxidant	x			
Anemia	x			
Anxiety				x
Appetite increase	x			x
Arthritis	x			x
Astringent		x		x
Bug bites/bee stings	x		x	
Blisters	x		x	
Cancer				x
Cholesterol	x			x
Cold	x			x
Constipation	x			x
Dementia	x	x		
Detoxification	x	x		x
Diabetes	x			x
Diuretic	x	x		
Dry skin	x	x	x	
Eczema	x	x	x	
Edema	x	x		
Emollient		x		x
Eye strain/poor night vision		x	x	x
Female reproductive support	x			x
Gallbladder support	x			x
Gallstones	x			x
Gas	x			x
Gout	x			x
Hepatitis B & C				x

	Leaves	Flowers	Stems	Roots
High blood pressure	X	X		
Infection prevention	X			X
Inflammation	X	X		
Influenza				X
Irritability				X
Jaundice				X
Joint pain	X	X		
Kidney support	X			X
Kidney stones	X			X
Lactation (increased milk supply)	X			
Laxative	X			X
Liver support				X
Mastitis	X			X
Menopause				X
Non-alcoholic fatty liver disease				X
PMS				X
Pre-diabetes				X
Scrapes and cuts	X		X	
Sore muscles	X	X		
Speed healing	X			X
Strengthen immune system	X			X
Stress	X			X
Upset stomach	X			X
Urinary tract support	X	X		X
Wart removal			X	
Yeast infections	X			X

Actions

Herbalists have certain terms, called "actions," they use to describe the properties of plants for medicine. These are more useful than simply saying "this plant is used for..." because they provide an understanding of how the herb works in the body.

Leaf:
alterative
anodyne
antacid
antilithic
antioxidant
antirheumatic
aperient
astringent
bitter
choleric
decongestant
depurative
digestive
diuretic
febrifuge
galactagogue
hepatic
hypotensive
immune stimulant
laxative (mild)
lithotriptic
nutritive
restorative
stomachic
vulnerary

Flower:
anodyne
astringent
cardiotonic
emollient
hepatic
vulnerary

Stem:
antibacterial

Root:
alterative
anodyne
antibacterial
antifungal
anti-inflammatory
antirheumatic
aperient
astringent
bitter
cholagogue
choleretic
decongestant
deobstruent
depurative
digestive
discutient
diuretic
galactagogue
hepatic
hypnotic
immune stimulant
laxative (mild)
lithotriptic
nutritive
purgative
sedative (very mild)
stomachic

Constituents

In addition to actions, it is helpful to know the "constituents" or chemistry of the dandelion.

Leaf:
beta-carotene
bitter glycosides
calcium
carotenoids (including lutein and violaxanthin)
choline
folic acid
inositiol
iron
manganese
phosphorus

potassium
taraxacin
terpenoids
vitamin A
vitamin C
vitamins B1 and B2

Flower:
carotenoids (taraxanthin, a mixture of lutein, flavoxanthin, and chrysanthemaxanthin)
lecithin

Root:
asparagine
caffeic acid
calcium
choline
coumestrol
fatty acids (myristic, palmitic, stearic, lauric)
flavanoids (lutein, luteolin, flavoxanthin, violaxanthin)
gallic acid
glycosides
inulin
iron
lactupicrine
levulin
mucilage
pectin
phenolic acids (quinic, chlorogenic)
phosphorus
phytosterols
potassium

Some Herbal Medicine Basics

Teas: One of the simplest ways to take herbal medicine is through teas. However, to get the best medicine from dandelion tea, be sure to follow the recipe directions closely and always cover brewing tea with a saucer (or similar device) to help retain its medicinal properties.

Decoctions: These are similar to teas, but are used with tougher plant materials, like dandelion roots. Decoctions apply more heat to the plant and steeping time is longer.

Poultices: When an herb is applied directly to the skin, it's called a poultice. To be effective, crush or mash the herb first. Hold poultices in place with a simple cotton cloth or with medical gauze and tape.

Tinctures: Possibly the most powerful form of herbal medicine, a tincture is typically an alcohol-based extract of an herb. For alcoholics or children, tinctures may also be made with vinegar or glycerin, though alcohol does a better job extracting the medicine from the plant. Alcohol-based tinctures have a longer shelf life (about 3 years).

Capsules: This is a way to make homemade herbal pills. Capsules are either animal-based (from beef-based gelatin) or vegetarian (from poplar trees). They also come in a number of sizes. "0" is considered standard size and holds 500 mg of herb. "00" is recommended in this book and holds about 750 mg of herb. There is also size "1," "2," and "3," which are smaller (400 mg, 350 mg, and 200 mg). Capsules are frequently found at local health food stores, or online through herbal stores.

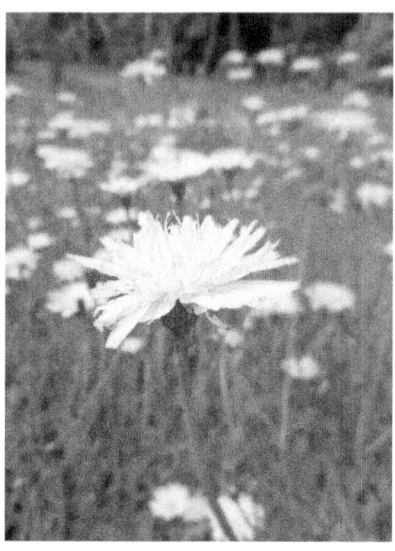

Dosage Guidelines

Alongside the recipes in this book, I've provided standard adult dosages. However, some additional insight may be required. For these guidelines, I've relied on the expertise of The Herbal Academy (TheHerbalAcademy.com), which offers many useful and free resources online.

Children's Dosages

There are different lines of thought about dosing children with herbal medicine; in particular, there are three respected guidelines, which go by the names of Clark's Rule, Young's Rule, and Cowling's Rule.

Clark's Rule:
child's weight divided by 150 = the fraction of adult dose herbalist should use when treating a child

Young's Rule:
child's age + 12 = X, followed by child's age divided by X = the fraction of adult dose herbalist should use when treating a child

Cowling's Rule:
child's age at next birthday divided by 24 = the fraction of adult dose herbalist should use when treating a child

Tips for Childhood Teas and Decoctions:

Infants: Even though dandelions are considered very safe for consumption (even by the skeptical FDA), there is a small chance of allergic reaction. Therefore, I wouldn't give dandelion to my baby, so I cannot recommend you give it to yours. Instead, it may be better if the mother consumes the dandelion medicine, and then gives her baby her breast milk.

Children 1 and up: Because children can be more sensitive to medication, always begin with the lowest dose possible. Watch the child for allergic reaction and to see how well the medicine is working. If it works well, there's no need to increase the dosage. If no symptoms of allergies appear, you may increase the dose slightly.

Tips for Childhood Capsules:

Infants and toddlers: Capsules are not recommended.

Older Children: Other forms of medicine are more suitable, since most children dislike swallowing pills.

Tips for Childhood Tinctures:

One of the most powerful forms of herbal medicine, tinctures are quickly absorbed into the bloodstream. They should be taken between meals and it's better to give several small doses a day, rather than 1 or 2 larger doses.

For children, always well dilute doses in water, milk, or juice. Start with the smallest dose, watch for effectiveness, and increase dose only if needed.

Senior's Dosages
Because seniors can be more sensitive to medication, herbalists give them smaller doses than they give other adults.

Over 63 years old: 1/3 of the standard adult dosage

Over 77 years old: 1/6 of the standard adult dosage

Tips for Senior Teas and Decoctions:

Begin with just 1 tea cup a day.

Tips for Senior Capsules:

Begin with 1 size "00" capsule 2 or 3 times daily. Avoid capsules altogether if there is any indication the patient doesn't swallow correctly.

Tips for Senior Tinctures:
Give several small doses a day, not fewer larger doses. Dilute tinctures in a small amount of water.

Standard Adult Dosages

Teas and Decoctions:
Up to 3 tea cups a day.

Capsules:
2 - 3 size "00" capsules up to 3 times daily.

Tinctures:
More powerful than most other forms of herbal medicine, and quickly absorbed into the bloodstream, tinctures should be taken between meals. It's better to give several small doses a day, rather than 1 or 2 large doses. Dilute tinctures in a bit of water.

For chronic illnesses, use 1/4 teaspoon - 1/2 teaspoon, 1 - 3 times daily.

For acute illness, use 1/4 teaspoon - 1/2 teaspoon, every 30 - 60 minutes until symptoms begin disappearing.

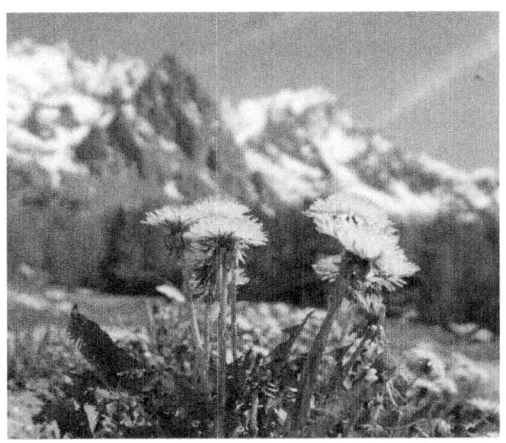

Contraindications
(Interactions and General Warnings)

All medicines - even those that are all natural - hold the potential for side effects. Though modern medicinal references (including the FDA) state dandelions are safe for most patients, it's smart to become aware of potential problems the plant could potentially cause. For professional advice on this matter, Master Herbalists, naturopaths, and Chinese Medicine practitioners are most helpful.

If you have ragweed allergies or are allergic to daisies, marigolds, or chrysanthemums, you should avoid dandelion. Some particularly sensitive people may even have a reaction to a mere touch of the plant.

Dandelion stems contain natural latex, which can cause contact dermatitis in some sensitive people.

Adequate scientific tests have not been conducted on dandelion use in pregnant and nursing mothers, so U.S. experts suggest these women do not consume the plant. (That said, many herbalists use dandelion to help relieve edema, anemia, and high blood pressure during pregnancy, and to increase milk supply after birth.) Consult your midwife or obstetrician for further advice.

If you are taking any prescription drugs, talk to your doctor before using dandelion. Because the herb is a diuretic (that is, it increases urine output), it can make prescriptions leave your body faster than desired.

If you are taking an antibiotic, dandelion root may decrease the effectiveness of the drug.

If you are taking lithium, do not also take dandelion, or a serious depletion of sodium may occur, due to excessive urination.

If you are taking a diuretic, use of dandelion could cause excessive urination, which could lead to depletion of nutrients.

If you are taking drugs to lower your blood sugar, it's theoretically possible the combination of dandelion and that prescription could make your blood sugar dangerously low.

If you are taking a medication that must be broken down in the liver, consult your physical before consuming dandelion.

If you are taking Cytochrome P450 (CYP) substrate drugs, dandelion will interfere with their absorption.

If you have a hormone-sensitive cancer, some experts suggest avoiding the use of dandelion.

If you have chronic kidney disease, do not consume dandelion; it can cause oxalates to accumulate in poorly functioning kidneys, leading to toxicity.

Although dandelion is an approved treatment for gallstones in European countries like Germany, if you have gallstones, it's recommended you consult your physician before consuming dandelion.

If you have obstructed bile duct, speak to your doctor before taking dandelion.

If you take blood-thinning medications (including aspirin), consult your physician. Some experts say dandelion might increase the risk of bleeding.

Some experts warn that dandelion may increase stomach acid, decreasing the effectiveness of antacids.

Never consume any wild plant without first positively identifying it.

Tips for Harvesting Dandelions

Buying Dandelions

Everywhere I've ever lived (including New York City) has dandelions in abundance, but some readers tell me they can't find wild dandelions growing in their area. Trust me when I say that's not a problem. We are fortunate to live in a time when wild food and medicine are making a come-back, and you can *buy* dandelions if you can't find them sprouting between the cracks in your sidewalk.

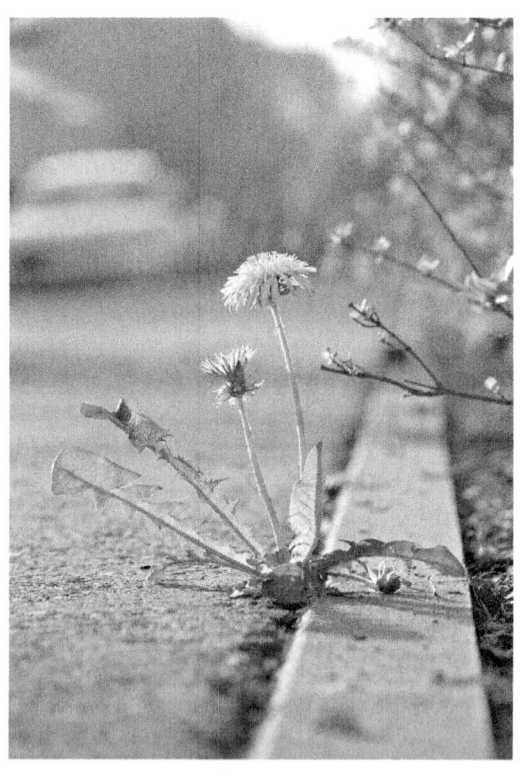

You may find fresh dandelion leaves at health food stores, farmer's markets, and upscale or gourmet markets. Or, you can look online for freeze dried (preferable, since this process retains more of the plant's nutritional value) or dehydrated dandelion leaves.

Dandelion roots are also easy to find online or in health food stores. They are dehydrated, typically, and sometimes roasted.

Dandelion flowers and stems are harder to find in stores and markets, but you can purchase dandelion seeds from online sources and popular seed merchants (like Johnny's Selected Seeds). Use these to plant your own dandelions in pots on your windowsill or balcony, or in a plot of ground in your yard. Never again will you have to worry about purchasing this valuable herb - though medicinally, wild dandelions tend to be more effective than cultivated ones.

Propagating Wild Dandelions

If you don't have dandelions in your yard, but find some public or wild source for them, it's relatively easy to propagate the plant for your own yard.

The most obvious way to do this is to collect the seeds:

1. Find a patch of dandelions that just went to seed, or cut some dandelion stems with flowers intact (preferably when the blooms are just beginning to wilt or turn brown); use string to tie the stems together and hang them upside down in a dark location (like a closet). Cover the flower end of the bundle with a brown paper bag. Wait for the flowers to turn to fluffy white seed heads.

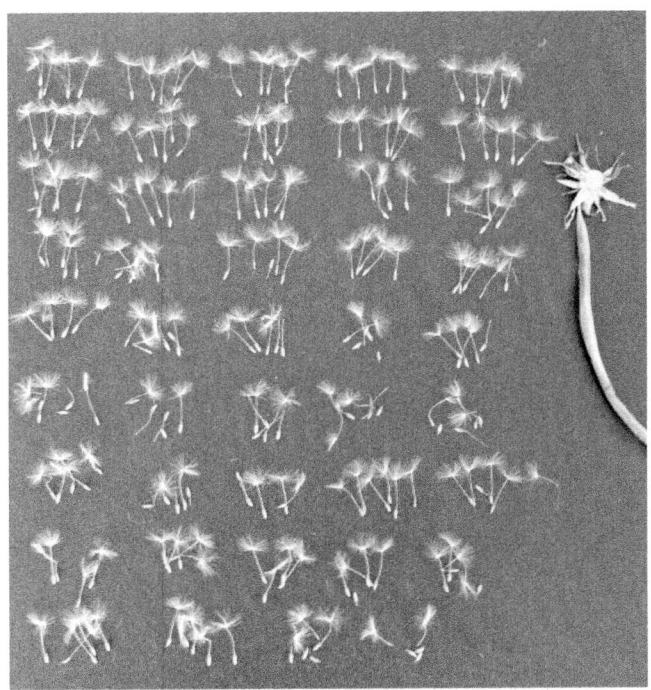

2. Snip off the seed heads and place them in a bowl.

3. Remove the seeds from the dandelion "fluff" and store the seeds in a jar kept in a cool, dark location.

To plant dandelion seeds:

1. In the early fall or early spring, stratify the seeds by keeping them in the refrigerator for 1 week.

2. Place the seeds on top of the soil, about 6 - 9 inches apart, assuming you want to grow full-sized plants. (If you just want to eat young dandelion leaves, you may sow the seeds closer together.) Do not bury the seeds, since they need light in order to germinate.

3. Lightly sprinkle a wee bit of soil over the seeds. Press down to ensure good contact between the seeds and the soil.

4. Gently water. Keep the seeds moist, but not damp. Seeds should sprout within 2 weeks.

TIPS:

- For less bitter leaves, keep your dandelion bed consistently moist.

- If growing dandelions in containers, use pots that are deep, since dandelions have a long root system.

To plant dandelion roots:

1. Dig up a large dandelion plant, using a dandelion puller or screwdriver, as described in the chapter "Dandelion Roots."

2. Break the roots into smaller pieces.

3. Plant the roots in soil, covering completely. Firmly press the soil over the roots. Water.

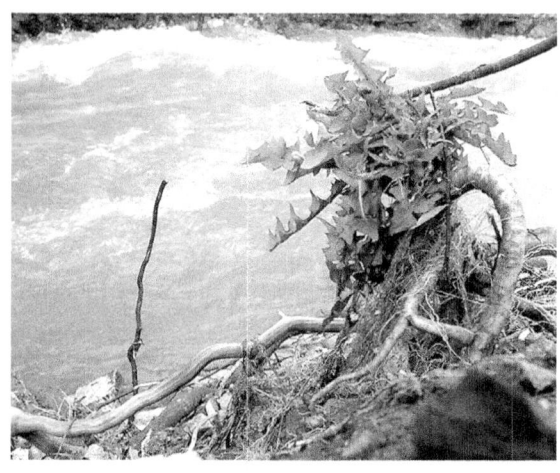

Picking Wild Dandelions

If you are able to find wild dandelions, they are preferable because they tend to have more medicinal properties than cultivated dandelions. Some well-meaning people may chide: "Save them for the bees!" But I assure you, dandelions are so abundant, the bees won't mind sharing with you.

However, when looking for wild dandelions, always follow three rules:

1. Never harvest dandelions near roadways (where the plants soak up chemical pollution) or from any location where chemical sprays (such as weed killers) may be used.

2. Never hoard the plant, and always leave behind more than you take. This ensures future harvests - and plenty left behind for wildlife.

3. Always positively identify any wild plant before eating it or using it for medicine.

Fortunately, dandelions don't have look-alike plants that are dangerous to eat. However, to ensure you're getting good medicine, make sure the plant has these key features:

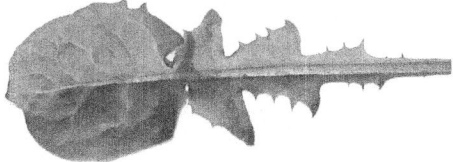

1. Tooth-shaped, hairless leaves.
2. Leaves and stems growing directly from the rootstalk in the soil.
3. One flower per stem.
4. Stems without branches on them.
5. A milky white sap when a stem is broken.
6. A thick root, looking rather like a small parsnip. Growing off this main root may be smaller, hair-like roots.

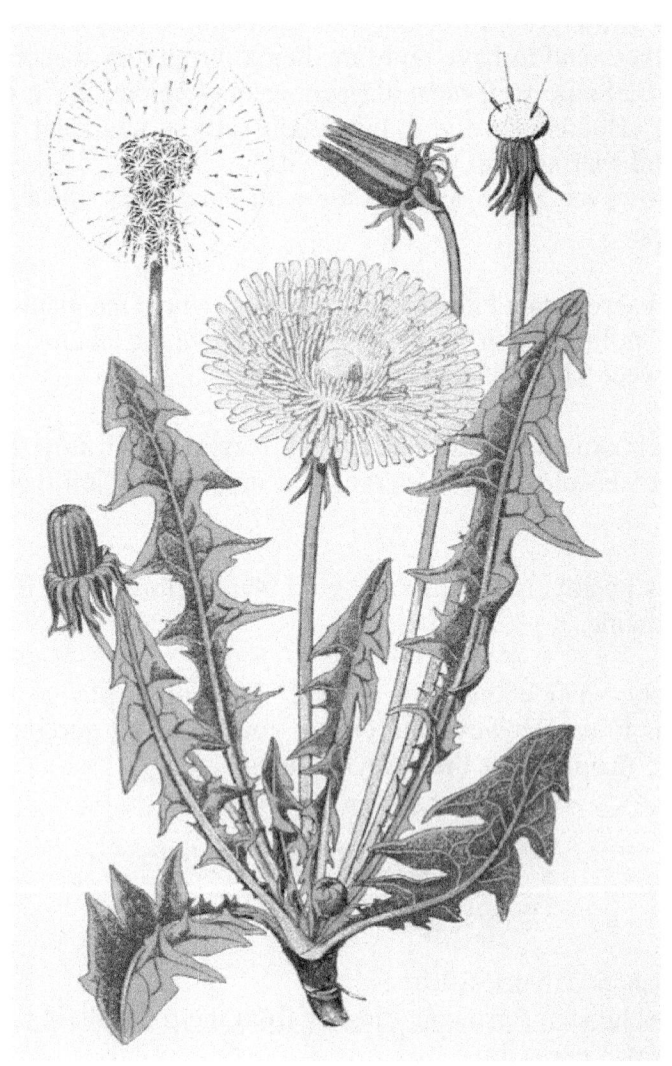

Dandelion Leaves

Acne, Alzheimer's, antifungal, antimicrobial, antioxidant, anemia, appetite increaser, arthritis, bug bites and bee stings, blisters, cold, constipation, dementia, detox, diabetes, diuretic, dry skin, eczema, edema, female reproductive support, gallbladder support, gallstones, gas, gout, high blood pressure, infection, inflammation, joint pain, kidney support, kidney stones, lactation, mastitis, scrapes and cuts, sore muscles, speed healing, strengthen immune system, stress, upset stomach, urinary tract support, yeast infections.

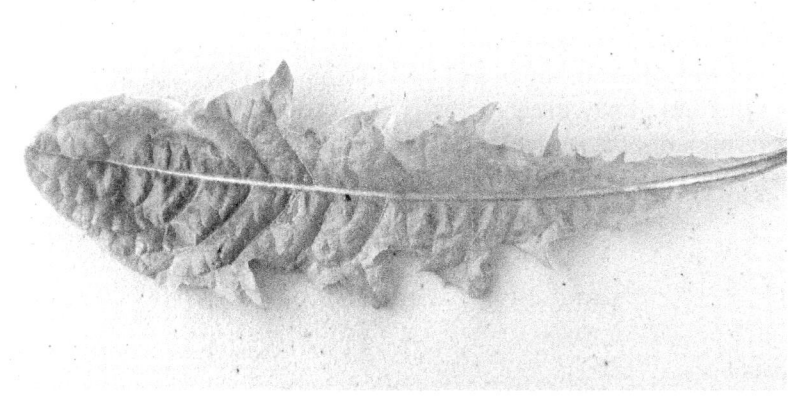

There's a saying that the best medicine is to eat well. I agree! When we eat nutritious food on a regular basis, we give our bodies powerful medicine to fight off illness and disease. One of the foods richest in nutrients is leafy greens; dandelion leaves fall into that category. But in addition to eating "dandy-leaves" (which I cover at length in *The Ultimate Dandelion Cookbook*), there are a number of easy ways to use the leaves as medicine.

Yes, some people might think it's strange to pick weeds from your yard and eat them or use them for medicine, but only a few generations ago, it was normal. Many families supplemented a thin Depression- or War-era diet with dandelion leaves, and during the 19th century, dandelion salad and medicine suggestions were found in nearly every household guide book. Before that, even the wealthiest considered choice weeds well worthy of their elegant tables and medicine cabinets.

Like spinach, kale, and collards, dandelion leaves are packed with nutrition. They are especially high in vitamins A, C, K, Omega 6, iron, phosphorus, potassium, and calcium.

Per Serving, Raw

	Dandelion leaves	Spinach	Kale	Collards
Calories	25	7	33	11
Carbohydrate	5 g	1 g	7 g	2 g
Protein	1.5 g	1 g	2 g	1 g
Vitamin A	5588 IU	2813 IU	10302 IU	2400 IU
Vitamin C	19.3 mg	8.4 mg	80.4 mg	12.7 mg
Vitamin K	428 mcg	145 mcg	547 mcg	184 mcg
Folate	14.9 mcg	58.2 mcg	19.4 mcg	59.8 mcg
Omega 3	24.2 mg	41.4 mg	121 mg	38.9 mg
Omega 6	144 mg	7.8 mg	92.4 mg	29.5 mg
Calcium	103 mg	29.7 mg	90.5 mg	52.2 mg
Iron	1.7 mg	.8 mg	1.1 mg	.1 mg
Magnesium	19.8 mg	23.7 mg	22.8 mg	3.2 mg
Phosphorus	36.3 mg	14.7 mg	37.5 mg	3.6 mg
Potassium	218 mg	167 mg	299 mg	60.8 mg

But, you may wonder, what do these weeds taste like? Sadly, some people have heard dandelion leaves are edible, run out to their yard, grab a leaf, and pop it into their mouth...only to spit the leaf out moments later. That's because there's a bit of art to eating dandelion leaves...unless you love bitter food.

The trick, then, is to start looking for dandy-leaves as soon as the snow melts, or as soon as several hard frosts have occurred. It's at this time dandelion leaves have their best flavor. Other times of the year, you can still eat dandelion leaves, but it will take a little more work to make them palatable food. The easiest method is to cook the leaves thus:

1. Bring a pot of water to a boil. Add the leaves and simmer for 1-2 minutes.

2. Taste. If the leaves still seem bitter, repeat with fresh water.

This method removes much of the bitterness, but also a small amount of the dandelion's nutrients. (Hint: Let the boiled water cool and use it to water your garden or house plants; just as dandelion leaves give humans good nutrition, the nutrients from those leaves also do a good job of feeding plants.)

For other ways to make bitter dandelion leaves palatable, please see *The Ultimate Dandelion Cookbook.*

Simple Ways to Preserve Dandelion Leaves

Because dandelion leaves are somewhat seasonal, I recommend preserving some for future use. They may be frozen, dehydrated, freeze dried, or canned. (Do bear in mind, however, that because dandelions contain a lot of natural moisture - which in turn contains many medicinal properties - when possible, it's best to use the plant fresh.)

Freezing: Fill a clean sink or large bowl with ice water. Fill a pot with water and place it over high heat. Bring to a boil. Add clean dandelion leaves and cook for 1 minute. Immediately drain and place the leaves in the ice water. Once the leaves are completely cool, pat them dry. Place in freezer bags. Freeze for up to 1 year.

Dehydrating: Place dandelion leaves on the trays of a dehydrator. (I prefer electric dehydrators because they dry herbs most efficiently - and at a temperature that retains their medicinal properties and nutrients.) Set the machine at 135 degrees F. and dehydrate until completely dry and crisp. Store in an air-tight container in a cool, dry, dark location. Alternatively, you may bundle leaves by the stems and hang them in a dark location, like a closet. Properly dehydrated leaves should be vivid green and last 1 or 2 years.

Freeze-Drying: If you are fortunate enough to own a home freeze dryer, simply place dandelion leaves on the machine's trays and process until no longer cold. Freeze dried leaves are delicate, so you may wish to powder them for storage. To store for 20 years or more, seal in a Mylar bag with an oxygen absorber.

Canning: If you like canned spinach or collards, you'll probably enjoy canned dandelion leaves. However, they are really only suitable as food-medicine. First, be sure you are completely familiar with safe pressure canning guidelines. (You can find guidelines on my blog: https://bit.ly/2wXK4rT)

You will need about 28 lbs. of leaves to make 7 canned quarts. Fill a pot with a steamer insert and a few inches of water. Place the leaves in the steamer and steam 3 - 5 minutes, or until completely wilted. If desired, add ½ teaspoon of salt to each canning jar. Loosely fill each jar with leaves and pour fresh boiling water over them. Leave 1 inch headspace. Process pints for 70 minutes and quarts for 90 minutes in a pressure canner.

Dandelion Leaf Tea

Aside from simply eating dandelion leaves as a cooked green, this is the easiest way to benefit from the medicine in the plant's leaves. Drink this tea as an anytime tonic, or use it if you're fighting a cold or infection, anemia, arthritis, high cholesterol or blood pressure, diabetes, edema or inflammation, gout, joint pain, or you need gallbladder or kidney support. If fresh leaves aren't available, you may use dried leaves; simply crumble and stuff leaves into both sides of a tea ball before placing it in a cup.

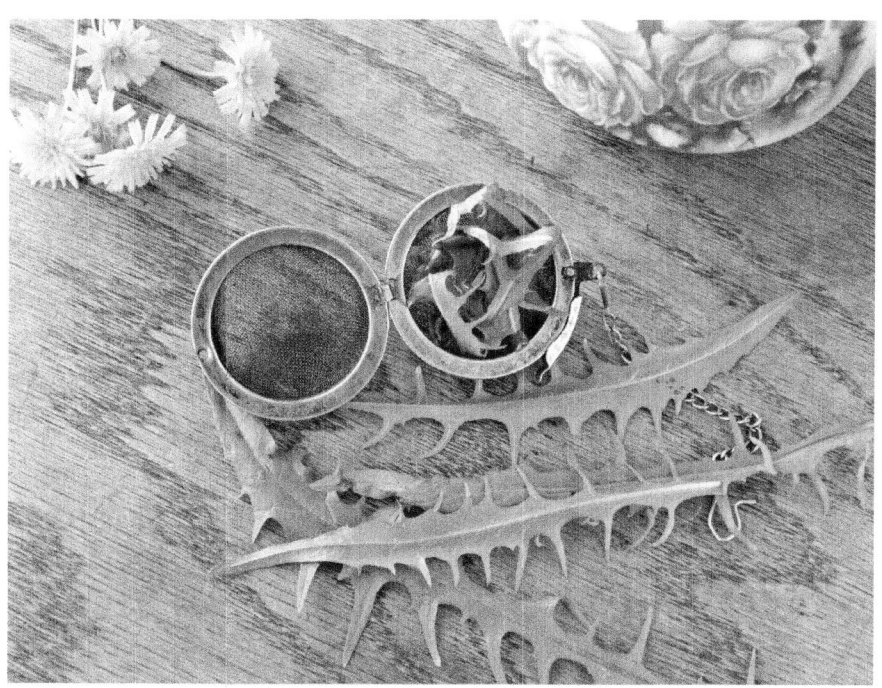

about 6 young, spring dandelion leaves, chopped coarsely
water

1. Place the prepared leaves in a tea cup and cover with boiling water. Cover the cup with a saucer until the mixture stops steaming, or about 10 - 15 minutes. The longer the steep, the stronger the flavor and the medicine of the tea.

2. With a small slotted spoon or a fork, remove the leaves and compost or otherwise discard them. If desired, you may sweeten this tea with real honey*. Drink warm or iced, up to 3 times daily.

* Some grocery store honey has added ingredients. Avoid this by reading ingredient lists carefully, or by purchasing honey from a local farmer.

Dandelion Leaf Vinegar

Enjoy this as a medicinal splash in your water, as part of a salad dressing, or in cooking.

fresh dandelion leaves
raw organic apple cider vinegar

1. Tightly pack a freshly washed glass jar with leaves.

2. Pour room temperature raw apple cider vinegar over the leaves until it comes nearly to the top of the jar. Secure a plastic lid* on the jar. Place in a dark location, like a pantry, for 6 to 8 weeks.

3. Strain through a fine sieve. (If desired, you may eat the "pickled" leaves. Otherwise, compost or otherwise discard them.) Pour into a freshly washed jar with a plastic lid* and store in a cool, dark location.

If you wish to use this vinegar strictly as medicine, take 1/4 - 1/2 teaspoon, 1 - 3 times daily.

* Vinegar reacts negatively with metal, so it's important to use a plastic lid.

Dandelion Leaf Poultice

Poultices are an ancient method of pulling infections or poisons from the body. You may find this poultice especially helpful for eczema, dry or itchy skin, rash (including poison ivy rash), psoriasis, or acne.

fresh or dried dandelion leaves
water

1. With freshly washed and dried hands, crush fresh dandelion leaves; alternatively, bruise and crush them gently with a mortar and pestle. Although fresh leaves are a better choice, you may also powder dried leaves in a coffee grinder or mortar and pestle.

2. To either fresh or dried leaves, dribble tiny amounts of water until you've created a paste. (Be sure dried leaves are completely rehydrated.)

3. Lay the paste over the affected area of skin. Cover with a piece of gauze held in place with medical tape or an elastic bandage. Or gently tie in place with a clean cotton cloth.

3. Apply a fresh poultice several times a day.

Variation 1: Use ice cold water to create a cold paste that helps dull pain and reduces inflammation.

Variation 2: Use hot water to create a hot paste that helps draw toxins from the area. To help keep the poultice hot, place plastic wrap directly over the paste. Use caution and make sure the poultice isn't so hot it will cause pain or injury when applied.

Variation 3: Instead of a traditional poultice, use medical gauze soaked in a long-brewed dandelion leaf tea (or a dandelion root decoction).

Dandelion Leaf Capsules

For convenience, or for patients who dislike the taste of dandelion leaves, it's easy to make capsules. You can find empty capsules on Amazon.com or at many local health food stores.

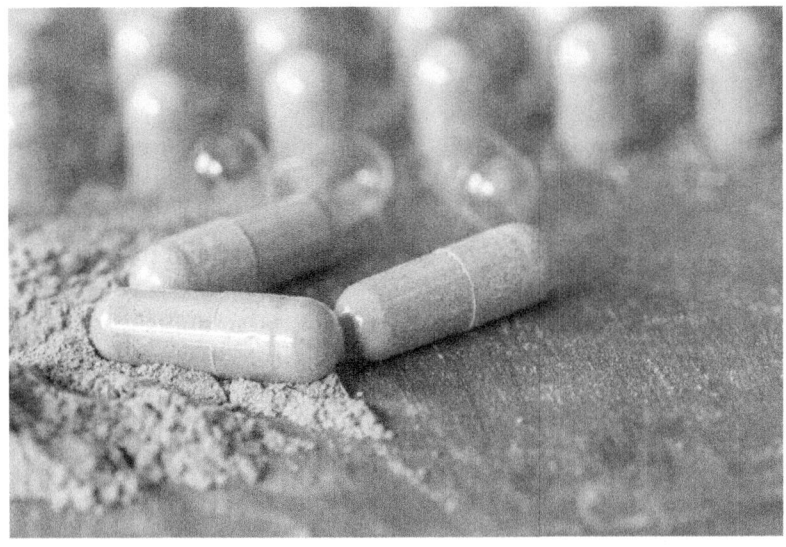

dried dandelion leaves

1. Powder dried dandelion leaves in a coffee grinder. Pour the powder into a bowl.

2. Scoop the powdered leaves into the longer end of a capsule. With the opposite hand, scoop more powder into the smaller end of the capsule. Work over the bowl so any excess powder falls into it.

3. Using gentle pressure, press both ends of the capsule together, sealing it. Repeat with remaining capsules, until all the powder is used up.

3. Store capsules in a glass jar with an air-tight lid in a cool, dark, dry location.

Adults may take 2 - 3 size "00" capsules up to 3 times daily.

Dandelion Leaf Juice

Dandelion juice was traditionally used for treating arthritis, kidney stones, night blindness, gout, hypertension, or simply as a nutritive or tonic. If desired, juice the leaves along with some fresh, chopped dandelion roots. 2 cups of chopped leaves results in about 1/3 cup of juice.

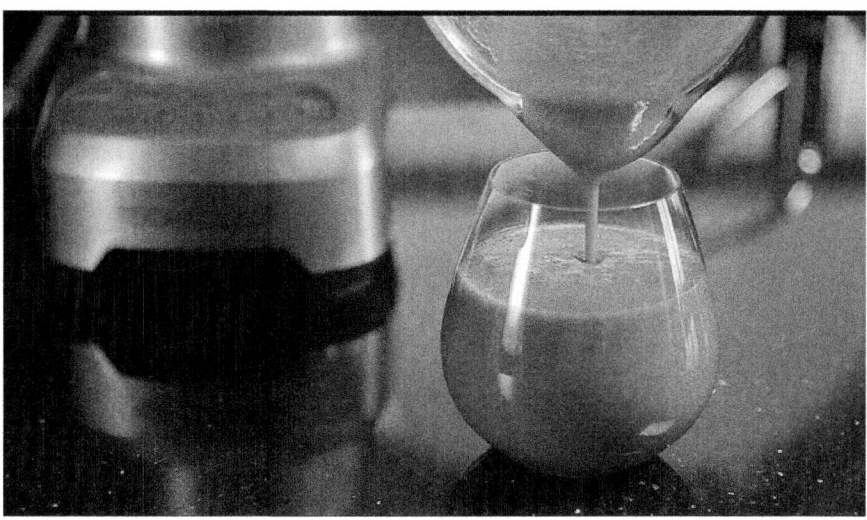

fresh spring dandelion leaves

1. Cut dandelion leaves into smaller pieces and run through an electric juicer.

Drink up to 6 tablespoons a day. Juice is most medicinal if consumed right away, but additional juice may be stored in the refrigerator in a glass jar with an airtight lid for up to 7 days.

Dandelion Leaf Bath

For women who tend toward yeast infections, dandelion baths may prove helpful. They can also aid dry or itchy skin.

fresh dandelion leaves

1. Cut a large piece of cotton fabric into a square. Place 1 or 2 handfuls of fresh dandelion leaves in the center of the fabric. Tie up the corners, turning the fabric into a closed ball.

2. Using a piece of string or ribbon, tie this ball over the spout of the tub.

3. Run hot water into the tub, making sure it passes over the bag. Squeeze the bag when you're done running the water, removing as much liquid from it as possible.

4. Allow the water to cool to a comfortable temperature. (For dry or itchy skin, make sure the water is no hotter than lukewarm.)

Alternatively, add pre-made (and cooled) dandelion leaf tea to the bath water.

Dandelion Leaf Oil (Slow, Traditional Method)

This oil is nutritive (meaning you can use it in cooking to add nutrients to your food), or may be applied directly to the skin to offer relief from soreness and joint pain.

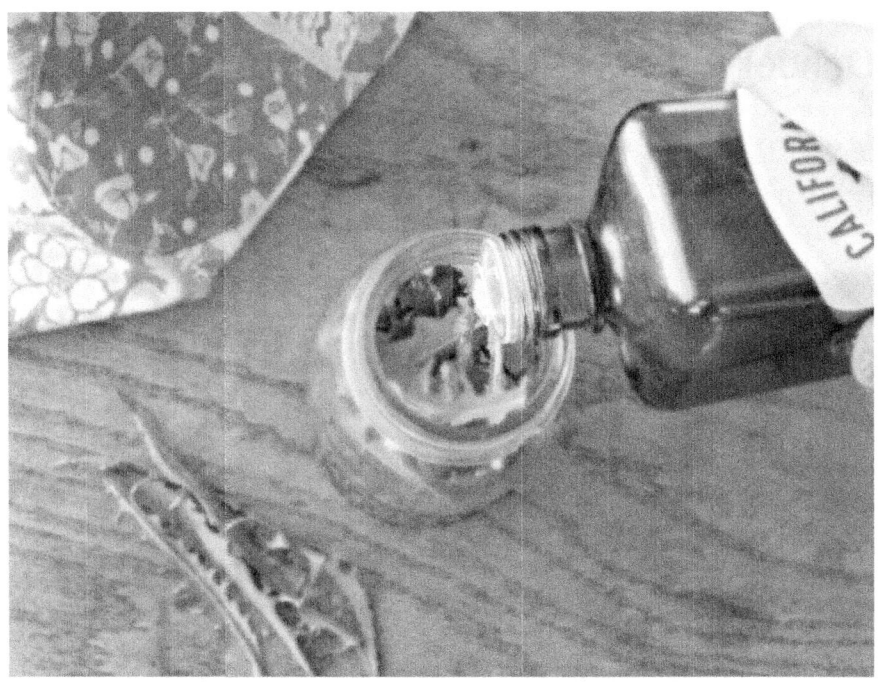

about 1 cup fresh, finely minced dandelion leaves
¾ cup olive oil

1. Spread the dandelion leaves onto a rimmed baking sheet and allow to air dry for about 1 - 7 days. This step removes some of the moisture from the leaves, which prevents the oil from becoming sludgy.

2. Fill a freshly washed glass jar half full with prepared leaves. Cover with olive oil, leaving 1/4 inch headspace at the top of the jar. Gently stir.

3. Put the lid on the jar and place it in a sunny location. Allow the mixture to steep for about 2 weeks, gently shaking the jar daily.

3. Strain through a sieve lined with coffee filters or two layers of cheesecloth. Compost or discard the solids. Pour the oil into a freshly washed glass jar with a well-fitting lid. Store in a cool, dark location and use within 3 weeks.

Dandelion Leaf Oil (Quick Method)

In a hurry? Use this method.

about 1 cup fresh, finely minced dandelion leaves
1 1/2 cups olive oil

1. Spread the dandelion leaves onto a rimmed baking sheet and allow to dry for about 1 - 7 days. This prevents the oil from becoming too moist and sludgy.

2. Add the prepared leaves and the olive oil to a small saucepan and gently bring to a very slow simmer. Barely simmer for 30 - 60 minutes.

3. Strain the leaves from the oil, using a fine mesh sieve. Compost or discard them. Pour the oil into a clean jar with an airtight lid and keep in a cool, dark location. Use within 3 weeks.

Dandelion Leaf Salve

Although dandelion flower salve is much more popular, a salve made with dandelion leaves may also prove helpful for joint pain, arthritis, and sore muscles. Look for salve containers at Amazon.com or a local health food store, or use jam-sized canning jars instead. This recipe makes about two 2 oz. jars.

3.5 oz of dandelion leaf oil
.5 oz of beeswax pastilles

1. Pour the oil and pastilles into a canning jar. Place the jar in a saucepan that's filled with several inches of water.

2. Place the pan on the stove, over very low temperature. Gradually increase the temperature until it's medium-low. Heat until the pastilles are completely melted.

3. Remove the container from the heat and pour the resulting salve into canning jars or salve tins.

Dandelion Leaf and Root Tincture (Folk Method)

Tinctures are considered one of the best ways to preserve herbs for medicine. Traditionally, dandelion leaves and roots were used together to make tinctures, though modern herbalists usually prefer to tincture the roots and leaves separately, since the roots take considerably longer to break down. You may chose either, using the method explained below. You can find tincture bottles at Amazon.com and at some local health food stores, or you may simply store your tinctures in glass jars with air-tight lids.

fresh dandelion leaves
fresh dandelion roots (optional)
80-90 proof vodka (or white or cider vinegar)

1. If using roots, separate dandelion roots from the leaves of the plant. Scrub roots well. Chop into small pieces.

2. Chop the leaves roughly. Alternatively, you may run the plant through a blender or food processor.

3. Fill a freshly washed canning jar with the prepared roots (if using) and leaves. With a wooden spoon, pack down the plant so there are no air pockets. Leave at least 1/4 inch headspace at the top of the jar.

4. Cover the plant with vodka, maintaining 1/4 inch headspace. Pack down the plant even more and add additional vodka. (You may substitute vinegar for vodka, but the finished product will not last as long on the shelf.)

5. Cover the jar with a sheet of wax paper. Over this, screw down the ring part of the lid. Shake the jar. Check the jar levels; if the mixture has more than 1/4 inch headspace, add more vodka.

6. Label and date the jar, then place it in a cool, dark location for about 6 weeks, shaking the jar at least once a week. When all the liquid in the jar has taken on color and tastes like the herb, the macerating stage is complete.

7. Strain the tincture: Place a fine mesh strainer covered with cheesecloth over a glass bowl. Pour the contents of the canning jar over the strainer and press the dandelion pieces to squeeze out all the liquid. Compost or otherwise discard the solids, retaining only the liquid.

8. Using a funnel, pour the strained liquid into a freshly washed glass jar or tincture bottle. Label with the date and type of tincture, and store in a cool, dry location.

Adults may take 1/4 teaspoon - 1/2 teaspoon, diluted in a little water, 3 to 5 times day.

Dandelion Leaf Tincture (Ratio Method)

The ratio method is the one professional herbalists use to create consistently potent tinctures. For dandelion leaves, I recommend a 1:1 ratio (equal parts leaves and vodka).

fresh dandelion leaves
80-90 proof vodka (or white or cider vinegar)

1. Chop the leaves into small pieces. Weigh them in grams.

2. Fill a freshly washed glass jar with the prepared leaves. With a wooden spoon, pack down the plant so it's well stuffed in the jar. Leave 1/4 inch headspace at the top of the jar.

3. Cover the leaves with an equal amount of vodka (measured in millilitres), maintaining headspace.

4. Cover the jar with a sheet of wax paper. Over this, screw down the ring part of the lid. Shake the jar.

5. Label and date the jar, then place it in a cool, dark location for about 14 days, shaking the jar at least once a week. When all the liquid in the jar has taken on color and tastes like the herb, the macerating stage is complete.

6. Strain the tincture: Place a fine mesh strainer covered with cheesecloth over a glass bowl. Pour the contents of the canning jar over the strainer and compost or otherwise discard the solids, retaining only the liquid.

7. Using a funnel, pour the liquid into a freshly washed glass jar or tincture bottle. Label with the date and type of tincture, and store in a cool, dry location.

Adults may take 1/4 teaspoon - 1/2 teaspoon, diluted in a little water, 3 to 5 times day.

Dandelion Leaf Sauté

Dandelion leaves are good medicine when eaten as food. I recommend using this method, which applies less heat than some other cooking methods, and is therefore less likely to sap the medicinal properties from the plant. You will find many other recipes for dandelion leaves in The Ultimate Dandelion Cookbook. *This recipe serves 2.*

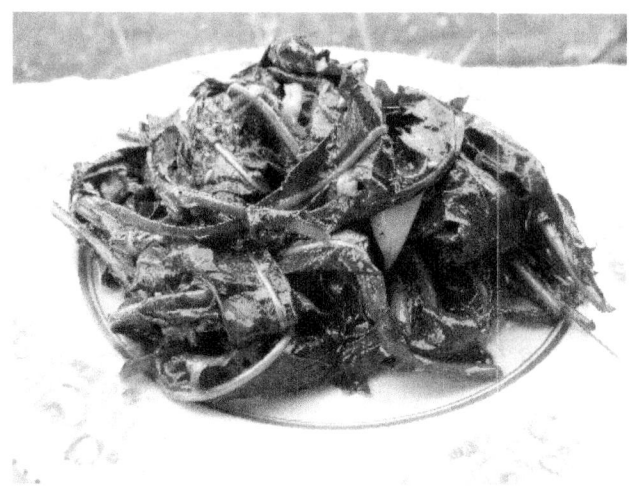

1 1/2 lbs. fresh dandelion leaves, coarsely chopped
1 tablespoon olive oil
1/4 teaspoon coarse sea salt
4 garlic cloves, minced
freshly ground pepper

1. Place a skillet over medium high heat and add the oil. Once warmed, add the garlic, sautéing until it barely starts turning color.

3. Add the dandelion leaves and season with salt and pepper. Cook and stir often until the leaves are bright green and wilted. Taste, adding more salt and pepper, if desired.

Variation: Cook a few strips of bacon in a skillet; drain the meat on paper towels and retain the drippings in the pan. Add the garlic, followed by the leaves. When the leaves are bright green and wilted, season, remove from the stove, and crumble the bacon on top.

Dandelion Flowers

Age spots, Alzheimer's, astringent, dementia, detox, diabetes, diuretic, dry skin, eczema, edema, emollient, eye strain and poor night vision, high blood pressure, inflammation, joint pain, sore muscles, urinary tract support.

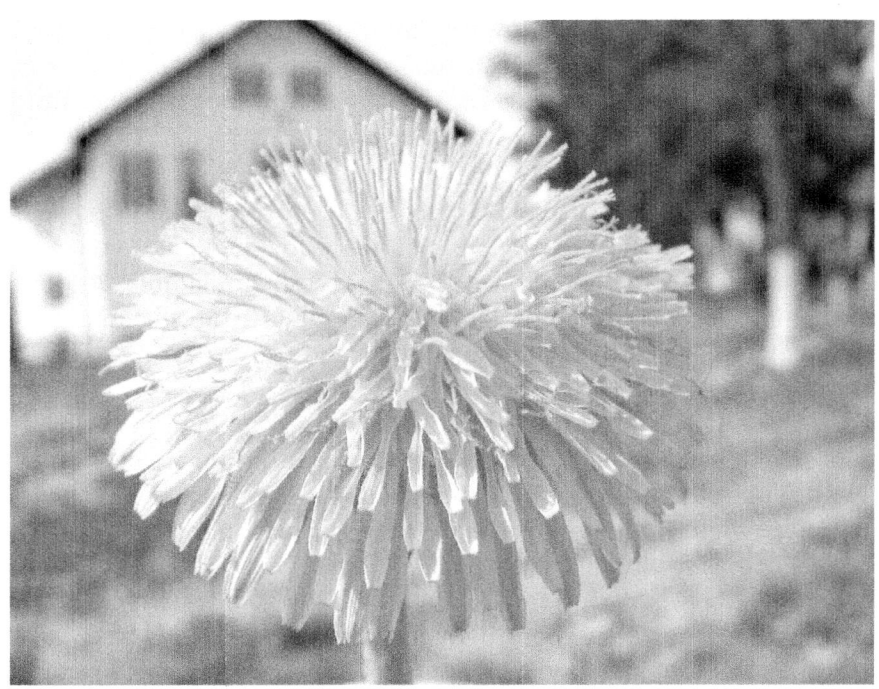

Even the casual observer can usually identify dandelion flowers growing in fields, lawns, and through cracks in the sidewalk. For the beginner, they are perhaps the easiest type of dandy-food and medicine, and are packed full of vitamins A, C, and B, beta-carotene, zinc, potassium, and iron. They also contain lecithin, a good tonic for the liver, which is also believed to maintain brain function and possibly slow or stop Alzheimer's disease.

Dandelion flowers have virtually no flavor all by themselves, although some people feel they have the slight taste of honey (a taste that's emphasized in old fashioned dandelion jelly). When cooked, the petals tend to take on the flavor of whatever they are cooked with. That said, the sepals (the green parts holding the petals together) are bitter; removing them, though, is a matter of preference.

When to Harvest Dandelion Flowers

Harvest dandelion flowers any time the plant is in bloom. I recommend using the newest blooms, snipping them off after morning dew has evaporated. Leave behind flowers that aren't fully opened, or that are beginning to wilt or turn brown.

Preserving Dandelion Flowers

When preserving dandelion flowers for medicine, you may either use a food dehydrator, a freeze dryer, or the freezer. (For medicinal purposes, when possible use the plant fresh, since more of the medicinal properties will remain intact.)

Freezing: After harvesting the flower heads, allow them to sit outside for a few hours. This lets any insects on the flowers crawl away. You may then lay the flower heads on a rimmed baking sheet and place them in the freezer; when they are stiff, transfer them to a freezer bag. Use within 1 year.

Dehydrating: For successful dehydrating, select flowers that have just opened. If you try to dehydrate older flowers, they will turn into white seed balls. Dehydrate the entire flower head in an electric dehydrator set at 95 degrees F., until completely dry and crispy. Alternatively, dry flowers on a mesh screen outside. If desired, remove petals after drying. Store in an air-tight container in a cool, dark, dry location and use within 1 - 2 years.

Freeze Drying: Lay flowers on the tray of the machine and process until they are no longer cold. Just as with dehydrating, older flowers might turn into seed puff balls. Store sealed in a Mylar bag with an oxygen absorber and use within 20 - 25 years.

How to Remove Dandelion Flower Petals

In my experience, the quickest way to remove dandelion petals from sepals is to hold the base of the flower in one hand and pinch the base of the flower head with the fingers on that hand. A gentle pull from the opposite hand will remove most of the yellow petals. You may also try rolling the base of the flower between your forefinger and thumb, which encourages the petals to fall off.

Another method is to hold the flower head in one hand and use scissors to snip off the petals at the base of the flower. Still another method is to hold the base of the flower with a strawberry huller and the petals of the flower with the opposite hand. Pinch and twist to remove the petals.

That said, I don't often bother removing the petals from the sepals. I find the slight bitterness of the sepals tasty in, say, dandelion flower tea.

Dandelion Flower Tea

This is the easiest method of enjoying the benefits of dandelion flower's medicinal properties. Drink this tea for urinary tract support, whenever you want a brain boost, to reduce joint pain and inflammation, or to help control high blood pressure.

fresh or dried dandelion flowers
water

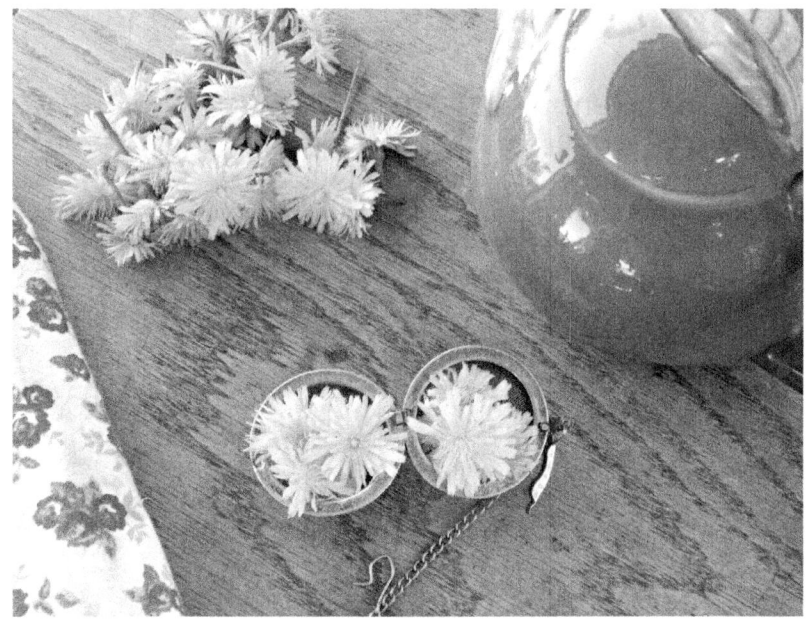

1. Pour some water into a small saucepan and place over high heat.

2. Pack fresh or dried flower heads into a tea ball. Close the ball and place it in a cup.

3. Once the water boils, pour it over the tea ball, into the cup. Cover the cup with a saucer until the tea stops steaming. Steep for 10 – 15 minutes. Drink warm or iced, up to 3 times a day.

Dandelion Flower Iced Tea

Adding some dandelion flowers to your favorite iced tea is an easy way to swallow your medicine!

fresh or dried dandelion flowers
water
1 - 2 black tea bags

1. Fill a quart jar about 1/3 of the way with fresh or dried dandelion flower heads.

2. Pour some water into a saucepan and bring it to a boil.

3. Pre-warm the jar (so it doesn't break when adding hot water) by carefully running hot tap water over the *outside* of the jar only. Allow the boiled water to cool a minute or two, then pour over the flowers, filling the jar. Add the tea bags.

4. Steep for at least 10 – 25 minutes, covering the jar with a saucer so no steam escapes. Strain, and serve the liquid over ice. Drink up to 3 cups a day.

Dandelion Flower Vinegar

Add a teaspoon of this vinegar to your drinking water, or use it on salads and in cooking. When you add a bit to your bath water, dandelion vinegar may also help relieve tired muscles. If you wish to take this herb vinegar strictly as medicine, take 1/4 - 1/2 teaspoon, 1 - 3 times daily.

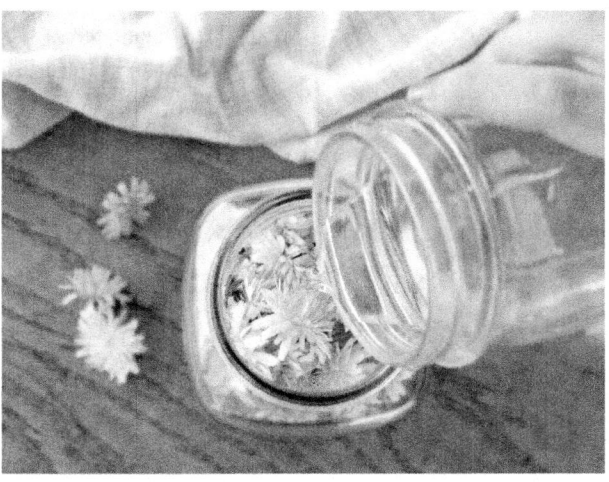

fresh dandelion flowers
apple cider or white wine vinegar

1. If using fresh flowers, lay them on a rimmed baking tray and allow them to sit at room temperature for 1 week. This removes some of the moisture from the flowers, which helps ensure successful vinegar.

2. Pack a freshly washed glass quart-sized jar with prepared fresh or already dried flower heads. Pour in enough raw apple cider or white wine vinegar to cover the flowers. Screw on a plastic lid* and keep the jar in a cool, dark location for 4 weeks.

2. Line a sieve with paper coffee filters or cheesecloth. Strain, composting or otherwise disposing of the solids.

3. Pour the liquid into a clean glass jar and cap with a plastic lid.*

* Metal lids react negatively with vinegar, so it's important to use a plastic one.

Dandelion Flower Oil (Slow, Traditional Method)

Use in any recipe calling for olive oil, or apply the oil directly to achy muscles and joints. This oil may also sooth dry, cracked hands.

> **1 cup fresh dandelion flowers**
> **¾ cup olive oil**

1. Spread the flowers onto a rimmed baking sheet and allow to dry for 1 - 7 days. This step helps prevent the oil from becoming sludgy.

2. Fill a freshly washed glass jar half full with prepared flowers. Cover with olive oil, leaving 1/4 inch headspace at the top of the jar. Gently stir.

3. Put the lid on the jar and place in a sunny location. Allow the mixture to steep for about 2 weeks, gently shaking the jar daily.

3. Strain through a sieve lined in coffee filters or two layers of cheesecloth. Compost or discard the solids. Pour the oil into a freshly washed glass jar with a well-fitting lid. Store in a cool, dark location and use within 3 weeks.

Dandelion Flower Oil (Quick Method)

In a hurry? Use this quicker method for creating dandelion flower oil.

1 cup dandelion flowers
1 1/2 cups olive oil

1. Spread the flowers onto a rimmed baking sheet and allow to dry for about 1 - 7 days. This prevents the oil from becoming too moist and sludgy.

2. Add the prepared flowers and olive oil to a small saucepan and gently bring to a very slow simmer. Barely simmer for 30 - 60 minutes.

3. Strain the flowers from the oil, using a fine mesh sieve. Compost or discard them. Pour the oil into a freshly washed jar with an airtight lid and keep in a cool, dark location. Use within 3 weeks.

Dandelion Flower Salve

This salve may be applied to the temples when suffering from a headache, or use it to soothe tired muscles and dry, cracked skin. For a salve that's more firm, slightly increase the pastilles; for a salve that's softer, slightly decrease them. Amazon.com and many local health food stores carry beeswax pastilles and salve containers, or you may store this salve in jelly jars. This recipe makes about two 2 oz. jars.

3.5 oz of dandelion flower oil
.5 oz of beeswax pastilles

1. Pour the oil and pastilles into a canning jar. Place the jar in a saucepan that's filled with several inches of water.

2. Place the pan on the stove, over very low temperature. Gradually increase the temperature until it is medium-low. Heat until the pastilles are completely melted.

3. Remove the container from the heat and pour the resulting salve into canning jars or salve tins.

Dandelion Flower Moisturizer

Combining two ingredients known for their skin-soothing capabilities, this simple moisturizer is good for dry skin brought on by cold weather and hard work. This recipe makes about one 4 oz. jar.

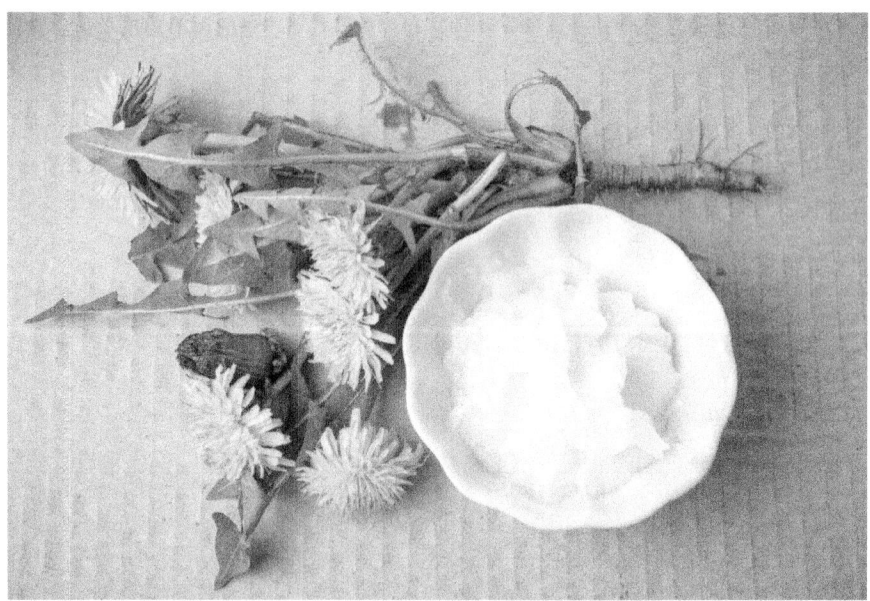

1/2 cup of coconut oil
1/4 cup of fresh dandelion flowers

1. Spread the dandelion flowers on a rimmed baking sheet and let them air dry for 7 days.

2. Place the prepared flowers inside a freshly washed canning jar. Place the jar in a saucepan that contains a few inches of water.

3. Slowly heat the saucepan, beginning on low heat and gradually increasing the heat to medium-low. Allow the jar to sit in the gently heated pan for 2 hours. Check the pan frequently to make sure the water doesn't evaporate; add more warm water, if needed.

4. Place a heat proof bowl under a sieve lined with a coffee filter or a double layer of cheesecloth. Carefully remove the jar from the pan and strain the mixture into the bowl. Refrigerate until the oil is firm again. Compost or otherwise discard the solids.

5. If desired, whip the moisturizer: Use a hand mixer to beat the oil for about 5 minutes, or until fluffy.

6. Spoon the moisturizer into small glass jars and store in a cool, dark location. (If your house is warm, store them in the refrigerator and bring to room temp before using.)

Dandelion Flower Lip Balm

If you tend to have dry, cracked lips, try this soothing balm. You can find beeswax pastilles, shea butter, vitamin E oil, and containers for packaging your finished product at Amazon.com or at some local health food stores.

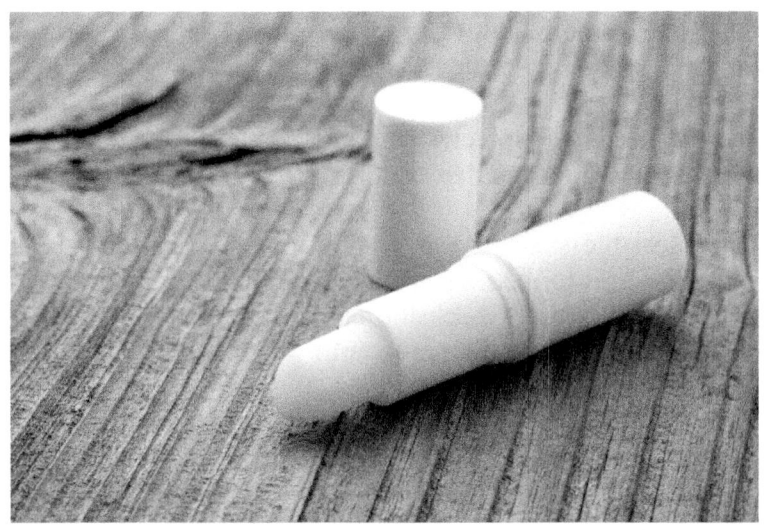

1 tablespoon beeswax pastilles
2 tablespoons shea butter
3 tablespoons dandelion oil
vitamin E oil

1. Pour the pastilles, shea butter, and dandelion oil into a canning jar.

2. Place a saucepan filled with a few inches of water onto the stove. Set the jar in the pan and, beginning with low heat, very slowly bring the heat to about medium. Allow the water to come to a gentle simmer. (Be careful; if you over heat shea butter, it becomes grainy.)

3. When all the ingredients are thoroughly melted, carefully remove the jar from the pan and stir in a drop or two of vitamin E oil.

4. Pour into lip balm containers and allow to sit at room temperature until the balm is firm.

This recipe is based on one found at ScratchMommy.com.

Dandelion Flower Bath Salts

Indulge in this healing bath remedy if you have dry skin or eczema, or simply want to refresh your skin.

> 1 3/4 cups pink Himalayan salt or other sea salt
> 3/4 cups Epsom salt
> 1/4 cup baking soda
> 3/4 cup powdered, dried dandelion flowers and/or leaves

1. To powder the dandelion, place dried flowers and/or leaves in a clean coffee grinder and pulse until fully powdered.

2. Combine all ingredients in a glass jar with a well fitting lid.

To use: Begin running the bath water. Once the bottom of the tub is covered with water, scoop a handful of the salt mixture into one hand and hold it under the running water. Use up to 2 handfuls per bath.

Dandelion Flower Water

In the 19th century, flower waters were extremely popular. Dandelion flower water was used to wash the face and is said to lighten age spots and freckles. It may also help prevent acne.

> fresh or dried dandelion flowers
> distilled water

1. Place about 1 cup of fresh or dried dandelion flowers in a non-reactive saucepan and cover with distilled water. Place the saucepan over medium high heat and bring to a boil.

2. Reduce the heat, cover the pan, and simmer gently for 30 minutes.

3. Strain through a fine sieve, pressing down on the flowers to get as much moisture from them as possible. Compost or discard the flowers. Allow the liquid to cool.

4. Pour the liquid into a glass jar, cover, and keep in the refrigerator.

To use: Splash face with the flower water, or apply to trouble spots with a cotton ball.

Dandelion Flower Bath

This easy bath water addition is soothing to the skin and mind.

dandelion flower water

1. Begin filling the bathtub. When the water fully covers the bottom of the tub, slowly add 1 - 2 cups of dandelion flower water.

2. When the tub is filled, allow the water to cool to lukewarm, if necessary.

Dandelion Flower Sugar Scrub

Dandy flowers are a natural emollient, meaning they soften and smooth the skin. Combine that with the moisturizing qualities of oil and the exfoliating qualities of sugar, and you have a truly natural beauty product.

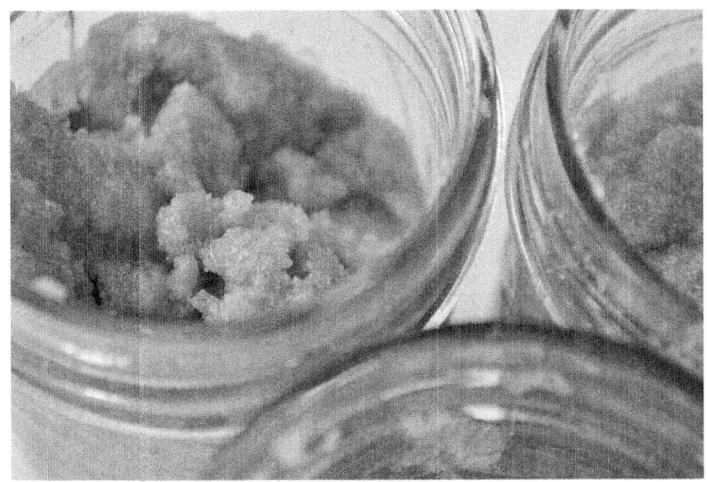

1/2 cup organic white or brown sugar
1/2 cup olive or coconut oil
1/2 cup powdered, dried dandelion flowers and/or leaves

1. To powder the dandelion, place dried flowers and/or leaves in a clean coffee grinder and pulse until fully powdered.

2. Stir all the ingredients together and spoon into a glass jar with an air-tight lid. Store in the refrigerator for up to 1 month.

To use: Scoop out about 1 tablespoon of the mixture and scrub over body while in the shower. Rinse well.

Dandelion Flower Lotion Bars

This is a creative way to apply dandy-moisturizer, and makes a unique gift. Beeswax and shea butter are available at Amazon.com and at many local health food stores. Check local craft stores for small soap molds, or buy them on Amazon. Even ice cube trays make good molds.

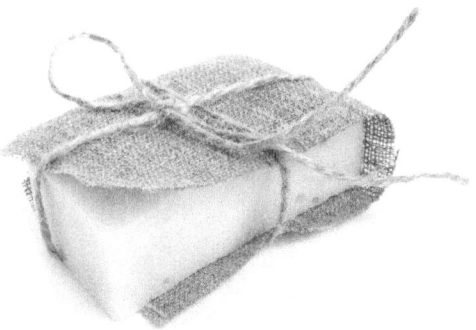

1/4 cup dandelion flower oil
1/4 cup beeswax
1/4 cup shea butter

1. Place all the ingredients in a canning jar.

2. Put a few inches of water in the bottom of a saucepan. Place the jar in the pan. Slowly heat the pan until the water gently simmers. Continue gently simmering until the ingredients are thoroughly melted. (Be careful; if you over heat shea butter, it becomes grainy.)

3. Pour the mixture into molds. Allow to thoroughly cool before popping the bars out of the molds. Store in air-tight containers.

To use: Warm a bar in your hands and run over dry skin. Body heat will melt the bar enough to leave behind moisturizer.

This recipe is based on one found at TheNerdyFarmwife.com.

Dandelion Flower Skin Serum

Dandelion flowers soften, smooth, and gently cleanse. Dandelion leaves help with acne and dry skin. By combining them with other soothing ingredients, it's easy to make you own, all natural face serum.

6 fresh dandelion flowers and leaves (alternatively, 1 tablespoon dried dandelion flowers and leaves)
½ cup aloe vera gel

1 teaspoon vitamin E oil

1. Pour the aloe, flowers, and leaves into a blender or food processor. Puree until the mixture is chunk-free and smooth. Pour the mixture into a bowl and allow it to sit at room temperature for about 1 hour.

2. Pour the mixture into a large square of cheesecloth. Bring up the corners, forming a bag, and squeeze the contents into a bowl. If necessary, strain again to ensure no plant particles remain in the gel.

3. Stir in the vitamin E oil.

4. Spoon the mixture into a glass jar with a well fitting lid. Store in the refrigerator for up to 3 months and use a clean spoon to dispense.

To use: Wash face, pat dry, and apply a small amount of serum to face and any other delicate skin areas. Allow to thoroughly dry before applying moisturizer.

Based upon a recipe found at TheHerbalAcademy.com.

Dandelion Flower Gelatin

This recipe combines the health benefits of dandelion flowers with those of gelatin. (Gelatin assists the liver, helps heal joints, and builds up skin, hair, and nails. It is also high in protein.)

**2 cups dandelion flower tea
2 tablespoons real gelatin (flavourless)
cane sugar, real honey, or Stevia to taste
turmeric (optional; for color)**

1. Pour the tea into a saucepan. Add gelatin and stir to combine.

2. Place the pan over medium heat and bring to a simmer. Gently simmer for 10 minutes.

3. Remove from the heat and allow to cool for a few minutes. (Watch the mixture carefully; if it sits too long, it will clump.)

4. Add sweetener, a little at a time, tasting as you go. Continue adding sweetener until you're happy with the flavor.

5. Spoon the gelatin into the squares of an ice cube tray or similar mold. You may also spoon and smooth into a 9 in. glass baking dish. Refrigerate overnight before serving.

Dandelion Flower Syrup

Syrups are a good way to get children to take their medicine. However, they are high in sugar; therefore use them sparingly.

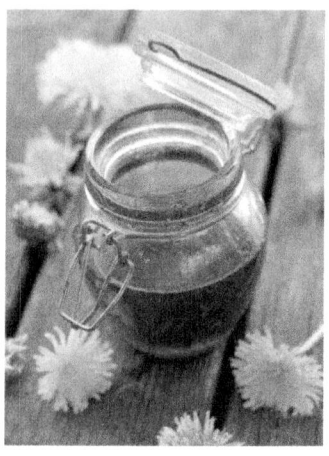

**2 handfuls fresh dandelion flowers
5 cups real cane sugar
lemon**

1. Pour 1 quart of cold water into a saucepan, add the flowers, and place over medium high heat. Bring to a boil.
2. Remove the pan from the stove and cover with a lid. Allow the mixture to sit overnight, at room temperature.

3. Strain the mixture through a fine sieve, composting or discarding the flowers. Retain the liquid.

4. Pour the liquid into a clean saucepan. Add the sugar and stir until mostly dissolved.

5. Cut the lemon in half and place one half in the sugar mixture.

6. Place the pan over medium high heat and bring to a boil. Reduce the heat and simmer until the mixture turns syrupy.

7. With a slotted spoon, remove the lemon and compost or discard it.

8. Pour the syrup into a glass jar with a lid. Store in the refrigerator.

Children may take 1/2 teaspoon - 1 tablespoon, 1 - 3 times daily.

Dandelion Stems

Antifungal, bug bites and bee strings, blisters, dry skin, eczema, scrapes and cuts, wart removal.

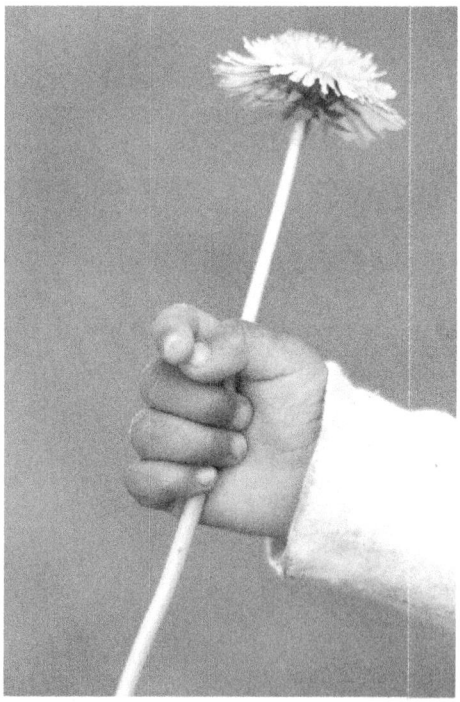

Perhaps the most neglected part of the dandelion is its stem. Although many children have enjoyed plucking a stem to remove the flower head and create a dandy "flute," few adults know the useful medicine those same stems provide.

The list of dandelion stem medicine isn't long, but that doesn't mean it isn't worthwhile. Do note, however, that this medicine is most effective when the plant is flowering.

Dandelion Stem Tincture

Although not frequently employed, dandelion stems may be added to whole-herb tinctures (see the chapter "Dandelion Leaves" for instructions).

Dandelion Stems for Minor Abrasions

Break open a fresh dandelion stem and squeeze its "sap" onto a scrape or cut.

Dandelion Stem Wart Removal

1. Break open a fresh dandelion stem and squeeze the "sap" onto a wart. Apply a bandage to help keep the medicine in place.

2. Repeat morning and evening until the wart is removed. Use a fresh bandage after each application.

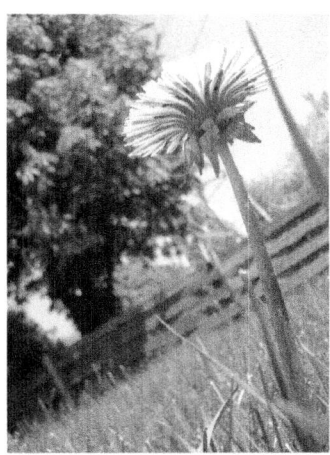

Dandelion Roots

Acne, Alzheimer's, antifungal, antimicrobial, anxiety, appetite increaser, arthritis, astringent, cancer, cholesterol, cold, constipation, detox, diabetes, emollient, eye strain and poor night vision, female reproductive support, gallbladder support, gallstones, gas, gout, Hepatitis B& C, infection, influenza, irritability, jaundice, kidney support, kidney stones, liver support, mastitis, menopause, non-alcoholic fatty liver disease, PMS, pre-diabetes, speed healing, strengthen immune system, stress, upset stomach, urinary tract support, yeast infections.

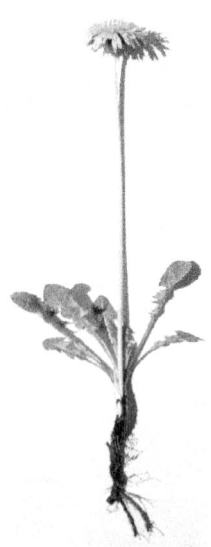

Perhaps the strongest dandelion medicine comes from the plant's roots, which are a great source of vitamins C, A, D, and B complex, beta-carotene, iron, potassium, zinc, biotin, phosphorus, and magnesium. They are also a good antioxidant.

In addition, dandy roots are notably rich in inulin, a prebiotic that encourages healthy microorganisms in the gastrointestinal tract and is widely considered a healthier carbohydrate for diabetics.

When to Harvest Dandelion Roots

When harvested in the spring, dandelion roots contain more sugar, making them sweeter to eat. In the fall, this sugar converts to inulin - a starchy substance used even in conventional medicine for high cholesterol and triglycerides, weight loss, and constipation. For this reason, and because the roots also use the spring and summer to store up nutrients the plant will require in the winter, fall is considered the best time to harvest medicinal dandelion roots.

How to Harvest Dandelion Roots

Dandelion roots are sometimes a challenge to dig up, so wait until the soil is moist - say, after a rain. (If no rain is in the forecast, use a garden hose to moisten the soil before digging.) Using a long screwdriver or a dandelion puller, insert the tool in the soil, near the base of the plant. Pull toward you. Repeat a few more times until you can pull up the plant. It will be difficult to get the entire root out of the soil - but that's fine. Leaving some of the root in the soil will ensure a new plant will grow in the old one's place.

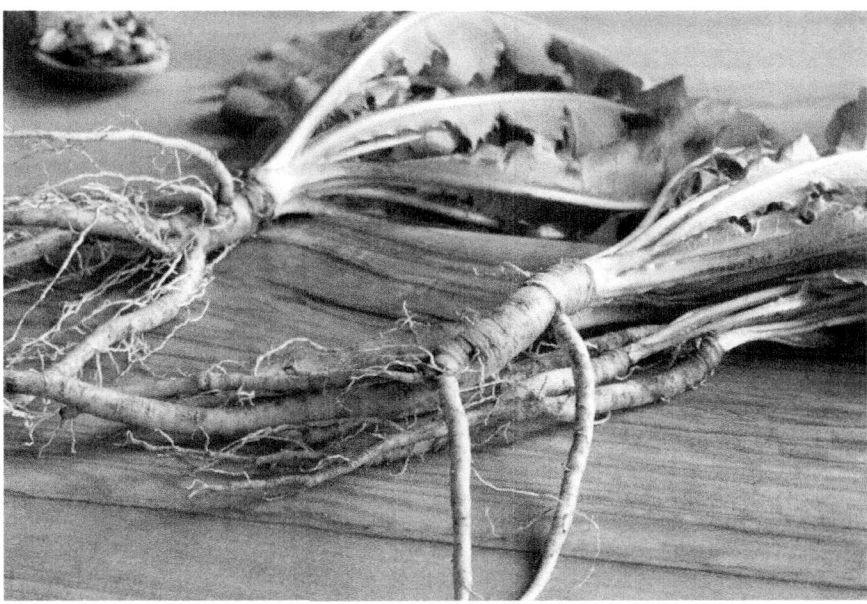

Preserving Dandelion Roots

Dandelion roots may be preserved by freezing, dehydrating, freeze drying, or roasting. (Directions for roasting are given in the "Dandelion Root Coffee" recipe in this chapter.)

Freezing: With a vegetable brush, scrub the roots well. Fill a clean sink or bowl with ice water and bring a pot of water to a boil. Boil the roots for 1 minute. (For roots that are large, chop first.) Immediately drain and dump the roots into the ice water. Once completely cool, drain well. Pat dry and place in freezer bags. Use within 1 year.

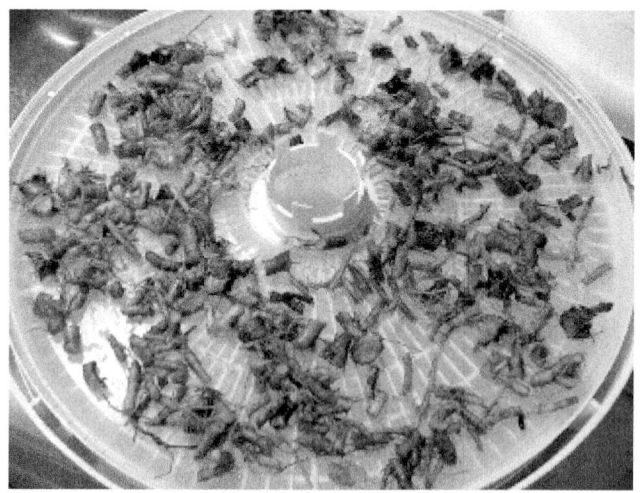

Dehydrating: Scrub the roots well, then chop into small pieces of about the same size. Fat roots should be halved, quartered, or sliced thin. Place on the trays of a dehydrator set at 135 degrees F. Dehydrate until there's no trace of moisture left. Allow to completely cool, then place in an air-tight container in a cool, dry, dark location. Use within 1 - 2 years.

Freeze drying: Scrub roots and pat dry. Chop into small pieces of about the same size. Place in the machine's trays and freeze dry until no longer cold. Store in a Mylar bag with an oxygen absorber for 20 - 25 years.

Dandelion Root Tea

For medicinal purposes, dandelion root is usually turned into some type of drink. Ideally, that drink allows you to digest some or all of the powdered dandelion root. This tea is especially good for liver function, anxiety, boosting the immune system, diabetes, female reproductive support and PMS, and gallbladder and kidney support.

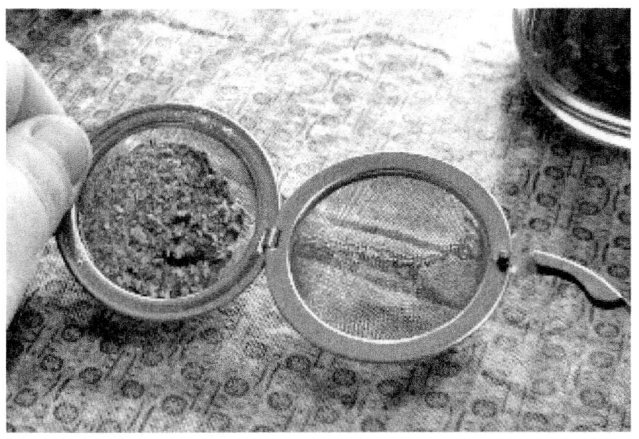

dried dandelion roots
water

1. Use a coffee grinder to at least partially powder dehydrated dandelion roots. Fill a tea ball with the roots and place the tea ball in a cup.

2. Pour boiling water over the tea ball. Cover the cup with a saucer, so steam doesn't escape.

3. Steep for about 10 - 15 minutes. The longer the steep, the more bitter the tea will be, and the higher its medical quality will be. Drink up to 3 tea cups a day.

Dandelion Root Decoction

Decoctions are very similar to teas, except they use more heat to draw out the medicinal properties of tougher materials, like roots.

fresh or dried dandelion roots
water

1. Place about 1 oz. of dried dandelion roots (or 2 oz. of fresh dandelion roots) into a saucepan. Add 2 cups of water.

2. Bring to a boil. Cover and simmer for 30 minutes.

3. Strain through a fine sieve lined in coffee filters or a double layer of cheesecloth. Compost or discard the solids.

4. Allow the decoction to cool enough to drink.

Consume up to 3 tea cups a day. Store any extra in a freshly washed jar in the refrigerator and use within 1 week.

Dandelion Root Water or Orange Juice

This is a simple way to obtain the medicinal power of dandelion root. Using orange juice helps cover the flavor of the root, which some people dislike.

dried dandelion root
water or orange juice

1. Using a coffee grinder, completely powder dehydrated dandelion root until you have 1 - 2 tablespoons.

2. Pour the powder into a glass of water or orange juice. Drink up to 3 times a day.

Dandelion Root Coffee

Although dandelion root is more medicinal if it's not roasted, dandelion "coffee" (which is caffeine free) is tasty and still has medicinal value.

dried dandelion roots
water

1. Preheat the oven to 250 degrees F.

2. Place dehydrated dandelion roots in a single layer on a rimmed baking sheet. Put the sheet in the preheated oven, with the door left ajar.

3. Stir every 15 minutes until roots are shrunk, crunchy, and golden, about 2 – 3 hours. (You may pre-roast the roots, cool completely, and store in an air-tight container in a cool, dry, dark location.)

4. Grind the roasted roots in a coffee grinder.

5. Pour 1 cup of water into a saucepan placed over medium high heat. Add 1 heaping teaspoon (or more, according to personal taste) of powdered, roasted dandelion root.

6. Bring to a boil, remove from the heat, and cover. Steep for 1 - 3 minutes, depending upon how strong you want the "coffee." Strain through a sieve lined in coffee paper filters or cheesecloth, composting or discarding the solids. Drink the liquid hot or iced, up to 3 times daily.

Dandelion Root Juice

This old-timey medicine was once the pride of apothecaries and drug stores. If desired, juice some fresh dandelion leaves along with the roots.

fresh dandelion roots

1. Cut fresh, scrubbed dandelion roots into pieces of a size recommended by your electric juicer's manufacturer.

Drink up to 6 tablespoons a day. Juice is most medicinal if consumed right away, but additional juice may be stored in a glass jar with an airtight lid in the refrigerator for up to a week.

Dandelion Root Capsules

For convenience, or for patients who dislike the taste of dandelion root, it's easy to make capsules. Purchase empty capsules at Amazon.com or at a local health food store.

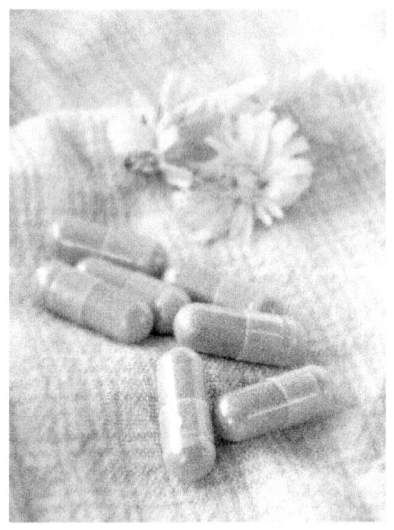

dried dandelion roots

1. Powder dried dandelion roots in a coffee grinder. Pour into a bowl.

2. Scoop the powdered roots into the longer end of a capsule. With the opposite hand, scoop more powder into the smaller end of the capsule. Work over the bowl so that any excess powder falls into it.

3. Using gentle pressure, press both ends of the capsule together, sealing it. Repeat until all the powder is used up.

4. Store capsules in a glass jar with an air-tight container in a cool, dark, dry location.

Adults may take 2 - 3 size "00" capsules up to 3 times daily.

Dandelion Root Vinegar

Although little used today, old herbals often contain recipes for dandelion root vinegar, which was used by the teaspoonful, medicinally. Some recipes do not call for heating the mixture, but I recommend it, to make a more potent medicine.

fresh dandelion roots
apple cider or white wine vinegar

1. Chop the dandelion roots finely and pour them into a freshly washed canning jar.

2. Cover the roots with vinegar, leaving about 1/4 inch headspace at the top of the jar.

3. Fill a saucepan with a couple of inches of water. Place the canning jar in the pan. Set the pan over very low heat and very gradually raise the heat to medium.

4. Watch the pan, making sure the water doesn't fully evaporate and that it never goes beyond a gentle simmer. Continue heating the jar this way for about 3 hours.

5. Carefully remove the jar from the saucepan and cover with a plastic lid*. Allow the jar to sit in a cool, dark location for 6 weeks.

6. Strain the vinegar, using a fine mesh sieve lined with cheesecloth of coffee filters. Compost or discard the roots. Pour the liquid into a clean jar with a plastic lid.*

Take 1/4 - 1 tablespoon, 1 - 3 times daily.

* Vinegar reacts negatively with metal, so it's important to use a plastic lid.

Dandelion Root Tincture (Folk Method)

Perhaps the best way to harness the power of dandelion root medicine is to turn it into a tincture. You can find tincture bottles at Amazon.com and at some local health food stores.

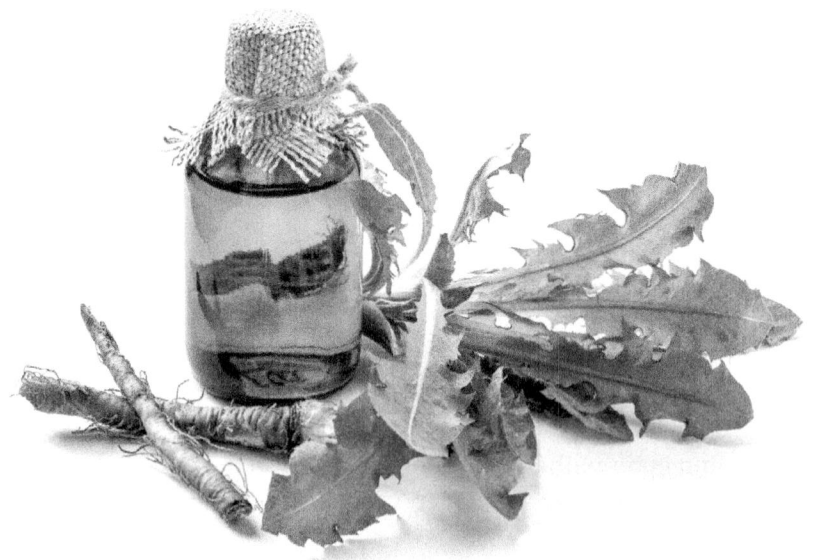

fresh dandelion roots
80-90 proof vodka, brandy, or whiskey

1. Slice gently scrubbed, fresh roots and slice into thin sections. Or, for a stronger tincture, run chopped roots through a blender. Place prepared roots in a freshly washed glass jar.

2. Cover the roots with vodka, brandy, or whiskey. Secure a tight lid on the jar. Label, including the date.

3. Allow the jar to sit in a cool, dark location for 4 - 6 weeks. Shake the jar every day.

4. When all the liquid in the jar has taken on color and tastes like the herb, the macerating stage is complete. Strain the mixture, retaining the liquid. Compost or discard the solids.

5. Pour the liquid into a freshly washed glass jar, or into a tincture bottle with a built in dropper. Store in a cool, dark location.

Shake the tincture before each use. (It's normal for a milkiness to develop at the bottom of the jar.) Adults may take 1/4 - 1/2 teaspoon, diluted in a little water, 3 to 5 times day.

Dandelion Root Tincture (Ratio Method)

This method of tincture making creates a more consistently potent medicine. I recommend using a ratio of 1:5.

> **fresh dandelion roots**
> **80-90 proof vodka (or white or cider vinegar)**

1. Scrub roots well. Chop and weigh the roots in grams.

2. Place the prepared roots in a blender or food processor and pulse until smooth.

3. Determine the amount of menstruum (liquid) appropriate for the tincture: Multiply the weight of the roots by 5. The answer is the amount of vodka to add, measured in millilitres.

4. Pour the vodka into the food processor or blender and pulse a few times.

5. Pour the mixture into a freshly washed glass jar and cover with a sheet of wax paper. Over this, screw down the ring part of the lid. Shake the jar.

6. Label and date the jar, then place it in a cool, dark location for about 14 days, shaking the jar at least once a week. When all the liquid in the jar has taken on color and tastes like the herb, the macerating stage is complete.

7. Strain the tincture: Place a fine mesh strainer covered with cheesecloth over a glass bowl. Pour the contents of the canning jar over the strainer and compost or otherwise discard the solids, retaining only the liquid.

8. Using a funnel, pour the liquid into a freshly washed glass jar or tincture bottle. Label with the date and type of tincture, and store in a cool, dry location.

Adults may take 1/4 teaspoon - 1/2 teaspoon, diluted in a little water, 3 to 5 times day.

A Sampling of Scientific Studies Supporting Traditional Dandelion Medicine Claims

Anticoagulant:

Yun SI, Cho HR, Choi HS. 2002. Anticoagulant from Taraxacum Platycarpum. Bioscience, Biotechnology, and Biochemestry. 66:1859-64

Anti-inflammatory:

Davaatseren M, Hur HJ, Yang HJ, et al. 2013. Dandelion leaf extract protects against liver injury induced by methionine- and choline-deficient diet in mice. Journal of Medicinal Food. Jan;16(1):26-33.

Jeon HJ1, Kang HJ, Jung HJ, Kang YS, Lim CJ, Kim YM, et al. 2008. Anti-inflammatory activity of Taraxacum officinale. Journal of Ethnopharmacology. February; 115(1):82-8.

Koh YJ1, Cha DS, Ko JS, et al. 2010. Anti-inflammatory effect of Taraxacum officinale leaves on lipopolysaccharide-induced inflammatory responses in RAW 264.7 cells. Journal of Medicinal Food. Aug;13(4):870-8.

Antioxidant:

Hu C,.Kitts DD. 2003. Antioxidant, prooxidant, and cytotoxic activities of solvent-fractionated dandelion (Taraxacum Officinale) flower extracts in vitro. Journal of Agricultural and Food Chemistry;51:301-10.

Choi UK1, Lee OH, Yim JH, et al. 2010. Hypolipidemic and antioxidant effects of dandelion (Taraxacum officinale) root and leaf on cholesterol-fed rabbits. International journal of molecular sciences. Jan 6;11(1):67-78.

Antibacterial:

Qian L, Zhou Y, Teng Z, Du CL, Tian C. 2014. Preparation and antibacterial activity of oligosaccharides derived from dandelion. International journal of biological macromolecules. 64:392-4.

O Kenny, N P Brunton, D Walsh, et al. 2015. Characterisation of Antimicrobial Extracts from Dandelion Root (Taraxacum officinale) Using LC-SPE-NMR. Phytotherapy research. Apr;29(4):526-32.

Katy Díaz, Luis Espinoza, Alejandro Madrid, et al. 2018. Isolation and Identification of Compounds from Bioactive Extracts ofWeber ex F. H. Wigg. (Dandelion) as a Potential Source of Antibacterial Agents. Evidence-based complementary and alternative medicine. Jan 1;2018:2706417.

Antidepressant:

Yu-Cheng Li, Ji-Duo Shen, Yang-Yang Li, et al. 2014. Antidepressant effects of the water extract from Taraxacum officinale leaves and roots in mice. Pharmaceutical biology. Aug; 52(8):1028-32.

Antifungal:

T I Odintsova, E A Rogozhin, I V Sklyar, et al. 2009. Antifungal activity of storage 2S albumins from seeds of the invasive weed dandelion Taraxacum officinale Wigg. Protein and peptide letters. Nov 1.

Antiviral:

Jia YY, Guan RF, Wu YH, et al. 2014. Taraxacum Mongolicum extract exhibits a protective effect on hepatocytes and an antiviral effect against hepatitis B virus in animal and human cells. Molecular Medicine Reports. April; 9(4):1381-1387.

Liu J, Zhang N, Liu M. 2014. A new inositol triester from Taraxacum Mongolicum. Natural Products Research. 28(7):420-423.

Zhongguo Zhong Xi Yi Jie He Za Zhi. 2000. Clinical and experimental study on antiviral activity of reduqing against human cytomegalovirus. Zhongguo Zhong Xi Yi Jie He Za Zhi. Apr;20(4):245-7.

Sidra Rehman, Bushra Ijaz, Nighat Fatima, et al. 2016. Therapeutic potential of Taraxacum officinale against HCV NS5B polymerase: In-vitro and In silico study. Biomedicine and pharmacotherapy. Aug 8; 83:881-891.

Yuan-Yuan Jia, Rong-Fa Guan, Yi-Hang Wu, et al. 2014. Taraxacum mongolicum extract exhibits a protective effect on hepatocytes and an antiviral effect against hepatitis B virus in animal and human cells. Molecular medicine reports. Apr; 9(4):1381-7.

Cancer:

Hata K, Ishikawa K, Hori K, Konishi T. 2000. Differentiation-inducing activity of lupeol, a lupane-type triterpene from Chinese dandelion root (Hokouei-kon), on a mouse melanoma cell line. Biological and Pharmaceutical Bulletin;23:962-7.

Choi JH, Shin KM, Kim NY, Hong JP, Lee YS, et al. 2002. Taraxinic acid, a hydrolysate of sesquiterpene lactone glycoside from the Taxacum Coreanum NAKAI, induces the differentiation of human acute promyelocytic leukemia HL-60 cells. Biological and Pharmaceutical Bulletin;25:1446-50.

Ovadje P, Hamm C, Pandey S. 2012. Efficient induction of extrinsic cell death by dandelion root extract in human chronic myelomonocytic leukemia (CMML) cells. PLOS one;7(2):e30604. doi: 10.1371/journal.pone.0030604.

Ovadje P, Chochkeh M, Akbari-Asl P, et al. 2012. Selective induction of apoptosis and autophagy through treatment with dandelion root extract in human pancreatic cancer cells. Pancreas. PANCREAS. Oct.;41(7):1039-1047.

Ovadje P, Ammar S, Guerrero JA, et al. 2016. Dandelion root extract affects colorectal cancer proliferation and survival through the activation of multiple death signalling pathways. Oncotarget. Aug 22. doi: 10.18632/oncotarget.11485.

Takasaki M1, Konoshima T, Tokuda H, et al. 1999. Anti-carcinogenic activity of Taraxacum plant. I. Biological and pharmaceutical bulletin. July; 22(6):602-5.

Chatterjee SJ1, Ovadje P, Mousa M, et al. 2011. The efficacy of dandelion root extract in inducing apoptosis in drug-resistant human melanoma cells. Evidence-based complimentary and alternative medicine. 2011:129045.

Ovesná Z1, Vachálková A, Horváthová K. 2004 Taraxasterol and beta-sitosterol: new naturally compounds with chemoprotective/chemopreventive effects. Neoplasma. February; 51(6):407-14.

Yasukawa K1, Akihisa T, Oinuma H, Kaminaga T, et al. 1996. Inhibitory effect of taraxastane-type triterpenes on tumor promotion by 12-O-tetradecanoylphorbol-13-acetate in two-stage carcinogenesis in mouse skin. Oncology. January; 53(4):341-344.

Sigstedt SC1, Hooten CJ, Callewaert MC, et al. 2008. Evaluation of aqueous extracts of Taraxacum officinale on growth and invasion of breast and prostate cancer cells. International journal of oncology, June; 32(5):1085-90.

Diabetes:

Hussain Z1, Waheed A, Qureshi RA, et al. 2004. The effect of medicinal plants of Islamabad and Murree region of Pakistan on insulin secretion from INS-1 cells. Phytotherapy research, Jan; 18(1):73-7.

Petlevski R, Hadzija M, Slijepcevic M, Juretic D. 2001. Effect of 'antidiabetis' herbal preparation on serum glucose and fructosamine in NOD mice. Journal of Ethnopharmacol. 75(2-3):181-184.

Detox:

Hfaiedh M1, Brahmi D1, Zourgui L1, et al. 2016. Hepatoprotective effect of Taraxacum officinale leaf extract on sodium dichromate-induced liver injury in rats. Environmental toxicology, Mar; 31(3):339-49.

M Gargouri, C Magné, I Ben Amara, et al. 2017. Dandelion-enriched diet of mothers alleviates lead-induced damages in liver of newborn rats. Cellular and molecular biology. Feb 28 ;63(2):67-75.

Diuretic:

Clare BA, Conroy RS, Spelman K. 2009. The diuretic effect in human subjects of an extract of Taraxacum Officinale folium over a single day. Journal of Alternative and Complementary Medicine. Aug;15(8):929-34.

Gallbladder:

Bohm K. 1959. Studies on the choleretic action of some drugs. Azneim-Forsh.9:376-378.

Hepatitis:

Jia YY1, Guan RF1, Wu YH1, et al. 2014. Taraxacum mongolicum extract exhibits a protective effect on hepatocytes and an antiviral effect against hepatitis B virus in animal and human cells. Molecular medicine reports.Apr; Apr ;9(4):1381-7.

Park CM1, Youn HJ, Chang HK, Song YS. 2010. TOP1 and 2, polysaccharides from Taraxacum officinale, attenuate CCl(4)-induced hepatic damage through the modulation of NF-kappaB and its regulatory mediators. Food and chemical toxicology. May 17;48(5):1255-61.

Park CM1, Cha YS, Youn et al. 2010. Amelioration of oxidative stress by dandelion extract through CYP2E1 suppression against acute liver injury induced by carbon tetrachloride in Sprague-Dawley rats. Phytotherapy research. Sept; 24(9):1347-53.

Kang JW1, Kim SJ, Kim HY, et al. 2012. Protective effects of HV-P411 complex against D-galactosamine-induced hepatotoxicity in rats. American journal of chinese medicine. Jun; 40(3):467-80.

Immune-enhancing:

Kim HM1, Lee EH, Shin TY, et al. 1998. Taraxacum officinale restores inhibition of nitric oxide production by cadmium in mouse peritoneal macrophages. Immunopharmacology and Immunotoxicology. Jun; 20(2):283-97.

Kim HM1, Oh CH, Chung CK. 1998. Activation of inducible nitric oxide synthase by Taraxacum officinale in mouse peritoneal macrophages. General Pharmocology. Feb; 60(1):61-9.

Yun SI1, Cho HR, Choi HS. 2002. Anticoagulant from Taraxacum platycarpum. Bioscience, Biotechnology, and Biochemistry. Oct; 66(9):1859-64.

Lee BR1, Lee JH, An HJ. 2012. Effects of Taraxacum officinale on fatigue and immunological parameters in mice. Molocules. Dec; 17(11):13253-65.

Influenza:

Wen He, Huamin Han, Wei Wang, Bin Gao. 2011. Anti-influenza virus effect of aqueous extracts from dandelion. Virology Journal. Dec; 8: 538.

Lipid lowering:

Liu YJ, Shieh PC, Lee JC, et al. 2014. Hypolipidemic activity of Taraxacum Mongolicum associated with the activation of AMP-activated protein kinase in human HepG2 cells. Food and Function. Aug;5(8):1755-1762.

Liver:

Davaatseren M, Hur HJ, Yang HJ, et al. 2013. Dandelion leaf extract protects against liver injury induced by methionine- and choline-deficient diet in mice. Journal of Medicinal Food. Jan;16(1):26-33.

Gulfraz M1, Ahamd D1, Ahmad MS1, et al. 2014. Effect of leaf extracts of Taraxacum officinale on CCl4 induced hepatotoxicity in rats, in vivo study. Pakistan journal of pharmaceutical sciences. 27(4):825-9.

Domitrović R1, Jakovac H, Romić Z, et al. 2010. Antifibrotic activity of Taraxacum officinale root in carbon tetrachloride-induced liver damage in mice. Journal of ethnopharmacology. Aug; 130(3):569-77.

Davaatseren M1, Hur HJ, Yang HJ, et al. 2013. Taraxacum official (dandelion) leaf extract alleviates high-fat diet-induced nonalcoholic fatty liver. Food and chemical toxicology. Aug;58:30-6.

Colle D1, Arantes LP, Gubert P, et al. 2012. Antioxidant properties of Taraxacum officinale leaf extract are involved in the protective effect against hepatoxicity induced by acetaminophen in mice. Journal of medicinal food. Jun;15(6):549-56.

You Y1, Yoo S, Yoon HG, Park J, et al. 2010. In vitro and in vivo hepatoprotective effects of the aqueous extract from Taraxacum officinale (dandelion) root against alcohol-induced oxidative stress. Food and chemical toxicology. Jun;48(6):1632-7.

Overviews:

Schütz K1, Carle R, Schieber A. 2006. Taraxacum--a review on its phytochemical and pharmacological profile. Journal of Ethnopharmacology. Oct 11;107(3):313-23.

González-Castejón M1, Visioli F, Rodriguez-Casado A. 2012. Diverse biological activities of dandelion. Nutrition Reviews. Sep;70(9):534-47.

Sweeney B, Vora M, Ulbricht C, Basch E. 2005. Evidence-based systematic review of dandelion (Taraxacum officinale) by Natural Standard Research Collaboration. Journal of Herbal Pharmacotherapy. 5(1):79-93.

Katrin Schütz, Reinhold Carle, Andreas Schieber. 2006. Taraxacum--a review on its phytochemical and pharmacological profile. Journal of ethnopharmacology. Oct 11; 107(3):313-23.

Women's Health:

Zhi X1, Honda K, Ozaki K, Misugi T, et al. 2007. Dandelion T-1 extract up-regulates reproductive hormone receptor expression in mice. International journal of molecular medicine. Sep;20(3):287-92.

Greenlee H1, Atkinson C, Stanczyk FZ, et al. 2007. A pilot and feasibility study on the effects of naturopathic botanical and dietary interventions on sex steroid hormone metabolism in premenopausal women. Cancer epidemiology, biomarkers and prevention. Aug;16(8):1601-9.

About the Author

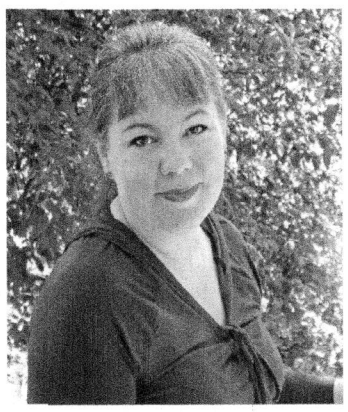

Kristina Seleshanko has a long obsession with herbal medicine, beginning with the planting of mint in her mother's garden (which quickly overtook the entire backyard). Today, Kristina enjoys wildcrafting, as well as growing cultivated herbs in her homestead garden. She writes for such magazines as *Woman's Day, Backwoods Home, GRIT,* and *Self-Reliance.* She is the author of 26 books, including the Amazon bestseller *The Ultimate Dandelion Cookbook.* She blogs about cooking, gardening, God, and more at **ProverbsThirtyOneWoman.blogspot.com**.

You May Also Enjoy...

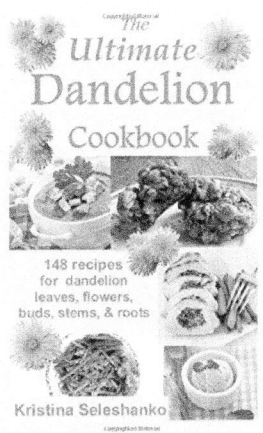

An Amazon #1 Bestseller!

Acknowledgements

Thank you, Suzannah Doyle, for always expressing eagerness about my creative projects, and for making this book better by offering thoughtful criticism. (Do check out her fun website, with lots of tips for musicians, at www.SuzDoyle.com.)

Thanks also goes to Melanie Miller, Kathy Barnett Walden, and herbalist Mark Allison, for volunteering to read a draft of this book and for giving their opinions about how I could make it better.

Photo Credits:
Oli Bac (8); Tia Monto (20); Fredrich Böhringer (23); J.D. Parker (25); Lamiot (26); Korn Vitthayanukarun (35); Breville USA (36); Pauh Nasca (44); Aleksandar Tomic (51); Koosen (52); Kim Love (55); Olga Popova (56); Madeleine Steinbach (63); Nadezhda Andriiakhina (70).

Index

Printed in Great Britain
by Amazon

44719708R00051